D1456803

The Healing Cell

The Healing Cell

How the Greatest Revolution in Medical History
Is Changing Your Life

Dr. Robin L. Smith
Msgr. Tomasz Trafny
Dr. Max Gomez

with a message from Pope Benedict XVI

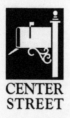

CENTER
STREET

New York Boston

Copyright © 2013 by Stem for Life Foundation
Quotation of the address of His Holiness Benedict XVI to participants in the International Conference on Adult Stem Cells: Science and the Future of Man and Culture (November 12, 2011) thanks to permission of the Libreria Editrice Vaticana (© Libreria Editrice Vaticana 2011).
The Pope's introductory and concluding remarks have been omitted.

Scripture quotations are from the New American Standard Bible®. Copyright © 1960, 1962, 1963, 1968, 1971, 1972, 1975, 1977, 1995 by The Lockman Foundation. Used by permission.

Center Street
Hachette Book Group
237 Park Avenue
New York, NY 10017

www.CenterStreet.com

Printed in the United States of America

RRD-C

First edition: April 2013
10 9 8 7 6 5 4 3 2 1

Center Street is a division of Hachette Book Group, Inc.
The Center Street name and logo are trademarks of Hachette Book Group, Inc.

The Hachette Speakers Bureau provides a wide range of authors for speaking events. To find out more, go to www.HachetteSpeakersBureau.com or call (866) 376-6591.

The publisher is not responsible for websites (or their content) that are not owned by the publisher.

Library of Congress Cataloging-in-Publication Data
Smith, Robin L., 1962-
  The healing cell : how the greatest revolution in medical history is changing your life / Dr. Robin L. Smith, Msgr. Tomasz Trafny, Dr. Max Gomez ; with a message from Pope Benedict XVI. -- First edition.
     pages cm
  Summary: "THE HEALING CELL is an easy to read, carefully researched, and clear-eyed view of medicine many decades in the making that is now paying off with treatments that repair damaged hearts, restore sight, kill cancer, cure diabetes, heal burns, and stop the march of such degenerative diseases as Alzheimer's, multiple sclerosis, and Lou Gehrig's disease. The emotionally and intellectually stimulating stories throughout the book dramatically illustrate that stem cell therapies can change the way we live our lives after being afflicted by a disease or trauma. The book is the result of a unique collaboration between the Vatican's Pontifical Council for Culture and the Stem for Life Foundation. It includes a special address by His Holiness Benedict XVI, urging increased support and awareness for advancements in adult stem cell research"-- Provided by publisher.
  Summary: "Stories of real health struggles of real people and the exciting scientific improvements and cures many of them are experiencing because of adult stem cell research and treatment." -- Provided by publisher.
  ISBN 978-1-4555-7292-2 (hardback) -- ISBN (invalid) 978-1-4555-7294-6 (ebook) 1. Stem cells--Popular works. 2. Stem cells--Research--Religious aspects--Christianity. I. Trafny, Tomasz. II. Gomez, Max. III. Title.
  QH588.S83S64 2013
  616.02'774--dc23
                              2012045650

You are a blueprint of divine,
A mirror reflecting his majestic design.
Seek inside whatever you desire,
For the universe is in you line by line.

> —*Rumi*
> *translation by Fred Nazem*

Contents

Contents

From the address of

His Holiness Benedict XVI

I would like to express the Holy See's appreciation of all the work that is done, by various institutions, to promote cultural and formative initiatives aimed at supporting top-level scientific research on adult stem cells and exploring the cultural, ethical, and anthropological implications of their use.

Scientific research provides a unique opportunity to explore the wonder of the universe, the complexity of nature, and the distinctive beauty of life, including human life. But since human beings are endowed with immortal souls and are created in the image and likeness of God, there are dimensions of human existence that lie beyond the limits of what the natural sciences are competent to determine. If these limits are transgressed, there is a serious risk that the unique dignity and inviolability of human life could be subordinated to purely utilitarian considerations. But if instead these limits are duly respected, science can make a truly remarkable contribution to promoting and safeguarding the dignity of man: indeed herein lies its true utility. Man, the agent of scientific research, will sometimes, in his biological nature, form the object of that research. Nevertheless, his transcendent dignity entitles him always to remain the ultimate beneficiary of scientific research and never to be reduced to its instrument.

In this sense, the potential benefits of adult stem cell research are very considerable, since it opens up possibilities for healing chronic degenerative illnesses by repairing damaged tissue and restoring its capacity for regeneration. The improvement that such therapies promise would constitute a significant step forward in medical science, bringing fresh hope to sufferers and their families alike. For this reason, the Church naturally offers her encouragement to those who are engaged in conducting and supporting research of this kind, always with the proviso that it be carried out with due regard for the integral good of the human person and the common good of society.

This proviso is most important. The pragmatic mentality that so often influences decision making in the world today is all too ready to sanction whatever means are available in order to attain the desired end, despite ample evidence of the disastrous consequences of such thinking. When the end in view is one so eminently desirable as the discovery of a cure for degenerative illnesses, it is tempting for scientists and policy makers to brush aside ethical objections and to press ahead with whatever research seems to offer the prospect of a breakthrough. Those who advocate research on embryonic stem cells in the hope of achieving such a result make the grave mistake of denying the inalienable right to life of all human beings from the moment of conception to natural death. The destruction of even one human life can never be justified in terms of the benefit that it might conceivably bring to another. Yet, in general, no such ethical problems arise when stem cells are taken from the tissues of an adult organism, from the blood of the umbilical cord at the moment of birth, or from fetuses who have died of natural causes (cf. Congregation for the Doctrine of the Faith, Instruction *Dignitas Personae*, 32).

It follows that dialogue between science and ethics is of the greatest importance in order to ensure that medical advances are never made at unacceptable human cost. The Church contributes to this dialogue by helping to form consciences in accordance with right reason and in the light of revealed truth. In so doing she seeks not to impede scientific progress, but on the contrary to guide it in a direction that is truly fruitful and beneficial to humanity. Indeed, it is her conviction that everything human, including scientific research, "is not only received and respected by faith, but is also purified, elevated, and perfected" (ibid., 7). In this way science can be helped to serve the common good of all mankind, with a particular regard for the weakest and most vulnerable.

In drawing attention to the needs of the defenseless, the Church thinks not only of the unborn but also of those without easy access to expensive medical treatment. Illness is no respecter of persons, and justice demands that every effort be made to place the fruits of scientific research at the disposal of all who stand to benefit from them, irrespective of their means. In addition to purely ethical considerations, then, there are issues of a social, economic, and political nature that need to be addressed in order to ensure that advances in medical science go hand in hand with just and equitable provision of health-care services. Here the Church is able to offer concrete assistance through her extensive health-care apostolate, active in so many countries across the globe and directed with particular solicitude to the needs of the world's poor....

I pray that your commitment to adult stem cell research will bring great blessings for the future of man and genuine enrichment to his culture. To you, your families, and your collaborators, as well as to all the patients who stand to benefit from your generous expertise and the results of your work, I gladly impart my Apostolic Blessing.

Foreword

Gianfranco Cardinal Ravasi
President of the Pontifical Council for Culture

There are thousands of scientific papers that discuss the search for medical remedies for disease, but most of them are written in the difficult-to-understand language of medical science. For this reason, I'm very glad that Dr. Robin Smith, Msgr. Tomasz Trafny, and Dr. Max Gomez have taken up the challenge to write this book, which clarifies recent scientific achievements in the field of stem cell research. Their work, a result of significant collaboration between the Pontifical Council for Culture and NeoStem, gave birth to an international conference, "Adult Stem Cells: Science and the Future of Man and Culture." That unique initiative emphasized that beyond scientific papers and academic debate, there are the patients—real people who have received significant benefits from ongoing medical investigation into stem cell therapies. They shared their experiences of suffering and successes on the path of healing. They are the primary protagonists of this book. However, behind their inspiring stories are doctors, scientists, and researchers whose efforts have overcome significant medical challenges, provided hope, and in many cases restored health.

More than ever, contemporary society is dominated by technological and scientific achievements. Each day brings news of new discoveries, and among these many branches of scientific investigation, those related to medical studies are of special interest to humankind. Medical science enables a better understanding of ourselves, which has led to numerous practical solutions to alleviate suffering stemming from age, sickness, and disability.

These developments are not only the domain of medical investigation. Today, the stage has been set not only for science but also for philosophical and theological anthropology and bioethics. Experts in these areas have painted a canvas of complex research in the field of regenerative medicine, and particularly in one of its most delicate nodes, that of stem cells. At the same time, there is an audience of people engaged in the pastoral field, in politics, in society, and in culture who seek guidance along a path in a land not yet fully explored, which is as fertile as it is fascinating and needs to be followed with care.

The Psalmist gives a surprising exclamation:

> I will give thanks to You,
> for I am fearfully and wonderfully made.
> *Psalms 139:14*

Certainly the human creature is marvelous at the level of conscience and thinking, and the same can be said of its corporeity and physicality. Classical Greek wisdom had this same intuition, and the philosopher Democritus of Abdera affirmed *ánthropos mikrós kósmos*: man is a microcosm. The understanding of the mystery of life is one of the most exciting and remarkable endeavors human beings can undertake.

The Healing Cell is a useful tool not only to discover a wonder of regenerative potentialities within our bodies, but also to explore how debilitating diseases can be overcome through courage, determination, intelligence, and new paths of investigation that lead to a better understanding of nature. This book brings hope to those who struggle with illness and encourages those who assist them—their relatives, friends, and loved ones—in a difficult battle. Today, studies on adult stem cells are a sign of hope that needs to be brought to public attention. The stories described in the following pages are special, and yet they are about common people, people like all of us, their lives broken down by infirmity and restored through careful and professional assistance. In the battle of saving lives, we can unite our forces and together help those who suffer.

The Church for centuries has played a crucial role in such efforts. For this reason, there is no antagonism between the Church and science, and in fact the two have been constant collaborators throughout the Church's two-thousand-year history. Catholic theologians have supported and contributed to scientific research and progress for centuries. It's a tradition that can be traced back to Saints Augustine and Thomas Aquinas, and it continues to yield exciting discoveries and treatments that benefit humankind. The current, contentious issue of stem cell technologies need be no different.

I invite those who have the privilege to read this book to not only read it with great attention, but especially to think about the major challenges humanity has faced in the previous centuries, the complexity of nature, and the moral and cultural influence of today's actions and decisions on future generations.

Introduction

Every generation witnesses a major revolution in one or more industries that changes the world forever. In our generation, it is the discovery of adult stem cells.

Most of us take our health for granted until we become ill, and then we realize just how precious health is and how many unfortunate people there are who suffer because they are not healthy. It's a long list. Each year, approximately fifty thousand Americans are diagnosed with Parkinson's disease. The Leukemia & Lymphoma Society estimated that in 2011, more than 1.5 million new cases of cancer were diagnosed in the United States. Macular degeneration is a common cause of blindness that affects about three million persons—a number that, according to the World Health Organization, is expected to double by the year 2020. We could cite statistics for many more serious illnesses, but you get the point.

This is a book about the real struggles of real people. But it's also a book about their strength, courage, faith, and, in many cases, their improvements or even cures because of adult stem cell treatments.

This book is also about the ethical science behind these successes and the hope this science presents for the people you'll meet in the following pages, the ones waiting desperately for cures—and who've lost precious time during their wait.

And so this is not an easy book, emotionally or intellectually. Be prepared for hard stories. But also be prepared for exciting science and, finally, for a clear-eyed view of medicine many decades in the making that is now paying off with treatments that repair damaged hearts, restore sight, kill cancer, cure diabetes, heal burns, and stop the march of such degenerative diseases as Alzheimer's, multiple sclerosis, and Lou Gehrig's disease.

These treatments aren't a science fiction author's far-fetched vision of the future. These are today's therapies, either currently used in hospitals or pushing their way through promising clinical trials.

The landscape of stem cell research and treatment is ever-shifting, populated not only by today's smartest, most motivated, and highly ethical scientists and doctors but also by hucksters, peddlers, and every brand of snake-oil salesmen. This book hopes to help you navigate the terrain by presenting facts, personal and scientific, from which you can draw your own conclusions about adult stem cell technologies.

Stem cell therapies can change the way we live our lives after being afflicted by a disease or trauma. This has already happened, continues today, and is going to revolutionize the world of tomorrow. Already, doctors have used stem cells to grow pouches and channels that replace bladders and windpipes, have used stem cells to grow new vessels that bring blood to dying tissue, and have coaxed stem cells into becoming liver tissue, insulin-secreting beta cells of the pancreas, and even cells that support a beating heart.

The somewhat premature claim that stem cells cure any disease obscures the very real fact that someday soon they actually might—and in some cases, they already have.

Take the case of Angela Harkson, a college freshman who one day woke up with numbness in her legs and then, by the end of the day, was numb from the neck down. Angela was diagnosed with multiple sclerosis and suddenly faced a world in which her health was slipping away. Then, five years ago, Angela had an adult stem cell transplant. Today, she is living a healthy, happy life.

Or Mark Cast, who in 1995 was diagnosed with chronic myelogenous leukemia. After eighteen months of chemotherapy but without a bone marrow match, Mark found himself in "blast crisis"—the end stage of the disease that carried a life expectancy of three to six months. After being turned away from a handful of clinics, Mark found Dr. Andrew Pecora, now chief innovation officer of the John Theurer Cancer Center at Hackensack University Medical Center and chief medical officer of the biotechnology company NeoStem, who got special permission from the Federal Drug Administration (FDA) for a one-time compassionate use of stem cells grown from the blood of a donated umbilical cord, which happened to be a close genetic match. From the small amount of stem cells contained in this umbilical cord, Dr. Pecora grew enough stem cells to reset Mark's immune system. Now, more than thirteen years later, Mark has lived to see both his children marry and is a proud grandfather of five.

In this book, there are many stories like Mark's and Angela's—many cases in which adult stem cell therapies have definitively saved or enriched lives. This book presents the facts of these stories, as well as the facts of the research and science behind them. This is a story with a beginning but no end in sight.

And because the beginning, it is said, is a fine place to start, let's start there: all the patients in the following pages and all the science in this book start with a single, magical cell—a stem cell that is the ultimate source of every human being and the later, adult stem cells that renew and maintain the body's tissues. Knowing how these first, magical stem cells give birth to the human body will help you understand how stem cell doctors reach back in this developmental time line to pluck the adult stem cells they need to protect and heal patients' bodies. Here is how these cells are born . . .

Like zipping closed a heavy winter jacket, twenty-three stick-like chromosomes from your father interlock in this first magical cell with twenty-three chromosomes from your mother to become the genetic blueprint for every subsequent cell in your body. The codes contained in this first cell will grow your skin and your bones and your blood. They will grow your cartilage and ligaments and tendons. They will grow your heart and your lungs. The patterns along the lengths of these twenty-three chromosome pairs will grow the 100 billion interconnected neurons of your brain.

Science calls this magical cell a zygote, but think of it as an architect given the green light for a massively complex construction project: you. If we would like to compare this enterprise to some image, perhaps the most convincing one would be building a house. It starts by bringing aboard birthing cells, or the well-educated general contractors that can do it all: in addition to steel and drywall, these very first cells can do electricity, plumbing, and all the other tasks needed to build your body. They're "totipotent," which you might recognize as being one small step down from the word *omnipotent*—these embryonic stem cells can build anything your body needs to grow and maintain itself.

Then, these totipotent embryonic stem cells make the construction project's first tough decisions, birthing four types of pluripotent cells. These are the subcontractors who specialize in steel (connective tissue), electricity (nervous tissue), sheathing and ducts (epithelial tissue), and the movement of elevators and machinery inside the building (muscle tissue). Here's the important part: each subcontractor gets a complete copy of the original blueprint—those twenty-three chromosome pairs—but they're instructed to build only certain parts. In pluripotent cells, huge swaths of the blueprint are redacted, scribbled out in black marker, so that these new pluripotent stem cells can see only the parts of the plan that are relevant to their jobs. For example, the pluripotent connective tissue stem cells retain access only to the parts of the blueprint for bone, blood, cartilage, lymph, and fat. The nervous tissue subcontractor knows how to build the nerves and neurons of your brain and spinal system, but nothing else.

It's not that they have any less genetic material than the original, totipotent cells; it's just that long stretches of this genetic material are silenced, colored over, leaving exposed only instructions for the projects for which these new, pluripotent cells have clearance. They can do a lot but not everything.

The cascade continues, and these pluripotent cells that can form many tissues delegate to underlings, and these underlings delegate, and their offspring delegate, until finally, far down the line, cells are specialized for one and only one function. Maybe a cell makes skin cells. Or maybe, even further down the line, a cell *is* a skin cell—it's no longer a stem cell that spits out tissue; it's the tissue itself. These lowest-of-the-low underlings form the vast majority of your body—they are your tissues, with the ability to do what they should do, but with very limited ability to renew themselves.

Again, even this lowly skin cell has the full construction blueprint—the two sides of the winter coat zipper that came together to form the original zygote from which all other cells in your body are born—but in a skin cell's genetic blueprint, all but the short length that details the functions of a skin cell is blacked out.

Now in your adult body, you have stem cells along the entire spectrum of specialization—some able to produce only one tissue type and others that keep their ability to make nearly any tissue type. Some of them are very special, like recently discovered "very small embryonic-like stem cells" or VSELs, which maintain all or almost all features of embryonic cells, but they exist in the adult body. Many researchers see these VSELs as a way to get pluripotency without the moral and ethical difficulties of embryonic cells and without the technological and tumor-forming challenges of induced pluripotent cells (or iPS cells; more on these below). Preliminary work, published in the journal *Stem Cells and Development*, described a population of VSELs isolated from the marrow of rodents that showed they differentiate into specialized cells to repair damaged heart tissue. An article in *Stem Cell Reviews and Reports* in 2011 described the potential role of these VSELs to repair damaged tissue in humans after a heart attack or stroke.

Alongside these stem cells, which again range from specialized for one tissue type to pluripotent VSELs, you have tissue cells themselves, which generally perform the function they're designed for, die, and are replaced. For example, the stem cells in the hippocampus region of the brain spit out new neurons that help you make memories, stem cells in your bone marrow crank out the components of your blood and immune system, and stem cells in your eye continue to ensure that you wake up each day with a new outer layer of tissue.

That's it. That's how from one special cell your body is made. Unfortunately, we damage our bodies in many ways. Take, for example, our skin. Because we do things like tanning, aging, or whacking our shins against car doors while trying to unload groceries, our skin cells die. Or take the case of Bobby Kenseth, who was born with epidermolysis bullosa, also called butterfly disease. It was as if the bit of Bobby's genetic blueprint that described how to make skin had gotten dirt on it. The smudged genes that told his body's workers how to make the skin protein keratin were defective, and without this keratin, Bobby's skin had no stickiness. It sloughed from his body with the slightest touch. Bobby Kenseth was as fragile as a butterfly.

After fulfilling his life's dream of flying in a glider, he said of the afterlife, "I think I'll be bored if the angels sit about on clouds plucking their harps all day. I'll be up there, getting them off their clouds, doing drops of one thousand feet, and then pulling up. I think you need to spice things up a bit." He died at age thirty-seven, in his wheelchair, of skin cancer stemming from his disease.

But what if we could have healed Bobby's defective blueprint? What if we could have taught his cells to make new skin? This is one promise of stem cell therapies.

At the Institute for Stem Cell Biology and Regenerative Medicine at Stanford University, researchers are working to grow skin that could permanently replace that of butterfly children. They do this by sampling a butterfly child's skin cells and clearing away the black pen that blots out the cells' potential to be anything, do anything. In other words, they reopen for business the genes that had been shut down as stem cells became skin cells. Then, they fix the faulty keratin genes and return these repaired, reinvigorated cells back to the patient's body, where these induced pluripotent stem cells can replant the blackened landscape with fresh, healthy tissue.

Or they will within a few years. Induced pluripotent cells require more research. Currently, the immune systems of laboratory animals tend to recognize these iPS cells as foreign and attack them. To work around these limitations, many researchers are studying other adult stem cells that don't require genetic manipulation. This includes VSELs, which exist in the adult body and so could be harvested, purified, and reinfused—and since VSELs are from a patient's own body, they are unlikely to trigger an immune system response. Other types of cells being studied by investigators include placental cells, which are believed by some to be immunoprivileged (they do not trigger the body's immune system); ELA cells, described by Parcell Laboratories as unique progenitor cells with unlimited therapeutic potential to facilitate the local repair of tissue; and versatile mesenchymal stem cells (MSCs), which are being studied as a potential "off-the-shelf" product in research medicine.

Again, this is the promise of stem cell research.

And almost universally, available and much of the stem cell therapies in development are derived from *adult stem cells*. Since many adult cells are able to create only a small, defined set of tissues, doctors can be more sure what these cells will make when they put them in patients. When we inject stem cells into the heart after surgery or stenting, we would like these cells to create new blood vessels and heart tissue. When we use stem cells to rescue a patient's immune system after obliterating it with chemotherapy and radiation as a treatment for leukemia, we want these stem cells to form the cellular components of the immune system. And when researchers inject stem cells into a three-dimensional collagen framework of a human bladder, we want the stem cells to generate cells that make up a bladder. (You'll read more about this exciting procedure in chapters 1 and 2.) It is much easier to get the tissue type you want from stem cells that are already specialized or semispecialized to create it.

According to a 2008 University of Pittsburgh McGowan Institute for Regenerative Medicine paper published in the journal *Cell Stem Cell*, these adult stem cells, capable of producing only a few tissue types in massive quantities, have been found "in multiple human organs including skeletal muscle, pancreas, adipose tissue, and placenta." It's long been known these adult stem cells are present in bone marrow. And according to the National Institutes of Health (NIH), they've recently been found in the brain, heart, liver, stomach, teeth, and elsewhere. Many researchers think that for any tissue in the body, there is a stem cell that generates it.

This use of adult stem cells also allows researchers to use a patient's *own cells*. Harvesting a patient's own cells is called "autologous" treatment, as opposed to "allogeneic" treatment, which obtains cells from a donor or another source outside the patient. Simply put, autologous adult stem cell treatments sidestep the huge difficulties of introducing foreign material into a patient's body, including the very real chance of rejection or destructive behavior.

So while the specifics of these techniques may sound like rocket science, the basic concept isn't: in most stem cell therapies, you can harvest adult stem cells that have the potential to create only one or a few types of tissue and so assure they will generate the tissue you want, without the tumor you don't. These adult stem cells are prepackaged for use.

We want to be clear and honest. The topic of this book is about science and medicine, but it is also about values, hope, religion, politics, and—why not?—about business, too. But in the end, it is about life and death. This book details the science and the successes of adult stem cell therapies. These successes are many, and they are powerful. These therapies can extend and enrich the lives of millions, perhaps billions, of people around the world.

Current therapies exist for many patients who needlessly suffer from curable diseases, and treatments are in the pipeline for people like butterfly child Bobby Kenseth. This book is for you and for your loved ones. These are stem cell therapies. In *this* generation, they may change your life.

Chapter 1

Organ Regeneration

On the twenty-fifth day of Katherine Manner's development in her mother's womb, something went wrong. Her spinal cord had grown normally, pushing down through what would become the bones of her back, but the sheath that holds the spinal cord failed to close. There was a hole. And as Katherine continued to grow, learning to kick when her mother listened to oldies and to roll when her mother drank coffee, her spinal nerves started to push through this tiny hole.

When Katherine was born, a small fluid-filled sac clung to the outside of her lower back, as if she'd been hit with a tiny water balloon. The diagnosis was immediate: spina bifida, a developmental disorder that affects about 1,500 babies born every year. It's an extraordinarily painful condition that left untreated can quickly lead to total paralysis below the spinal cord opening.

In the hours after her birth and diagnosis, surgeons closed the hole in Katherine's back and spine, carefully packing the nerves in through the hole and then closing it with a small patch of donated dura mater—the strong tissue that forms the sac around the brain and spinal cord.

But Katherine was far from being out of the woods. Cerebrospinal fluid is produced in the brain and flows down from the brain through the spinal system, providing nutrients and removing toxins. And, as is common in spina bifida, Katherine's cerebrospinal fluid wasn't circulating properly. Instead of gravity pulling it downward like a cleansing rain, this fluid was trapped in her skull, and as her brain produced more fluid, it pushed outward, creating constant pressure and headache. This is hydrocephaly, also called water on the brain, and in the past, at around age twelve when the skull couldn't grow anymore, the pressure of this cerebrospinal fluid would start to slowly squeeze the brain until it was all but destroyed. In 1900, life expectancy for a person with hydrocephaly was about twenty-one years. Luckily, surgeons again had an answer, inserting a long tube called a shunt that drained excess cerebrospinal fluid from Katherine's brain and released it into her abdomen.

As she learned to walk, orthopedic surgeons worked to correct the deformities in the bones of her spinal column. Katherine was fitted with arm-brace crutches that she would use for the rest of her life. And as she grew, neurosurgeons periodically adjusted the length of the tube draining fluid from her brain to her abdomen.

Katherine developed into a vivacious twelve-year-old with friends and big plans for the future. "I liked to talk on the phone a lot," she said. But spina bifida wasn't done with her yet. When the little bundle of nerves protruded from her spine, the lines of communication between Katherine's brain and her bladder had been disrupted, and after twelve years without nerves telling her bladder and pelvic muscles when to contract and relax, the lack of exercise turned muscle to leather, and the bladder lost its ability to hold liquid.

"If she drank a cup of water or a cup of juice, her bladder's pressures were at such an intense point she would have something called a bladder burst," recalled her mother, Tracy, in an interview with CNN. Katherine had to wear a diaper. But more importantly, this bladder burst also backed up toxic urine into Katherine's kidneys. As her middle-school friends worried about cliques and homework, Katherine and her family worried about renal failure.

And unfortunately this was the end of the line for existing medicine. Sure, patients in the past had rebuilt damaged bladders with grafts from their intestines, but "when you put a piece of intestine to function as a bladder, you start having absorption of things you shouldn't be having, and this may lead to problems with bone growth, mucus production, certain metabolic problems, even cancer," says Dr. Anthony Atala, head of the Institute for Regenerative Medicine at Wake Forest University and one of the leading authorities on pediatric bladder disease. Repair with intestinal tissue is a flawed fix. Katherine was on a road to kidney failure, dialysis, and a shortened lifetime hooked to a machine.

Traditionally, Katherine's best option was a kidney transplant. But according to UNOS, the United Network for Organ Sharing, an average of more than one hundred thousand people at any given time are waiting for lifesaving organ transplants in the United States, and because of shortages of available organs, seventeen patients die every day. Even with a new kidney, Katherine's damaged bladder would eventually destroy it as well.

But instead of throwing up their hands, calling kidney failure one of the things you can't change and praying for the courage to accept her condition, Katherine's family stepped beyond existing medicine's end of the line. They looked to the future and enrolled her in a first-of-its-kind clinical trial at Boston Children's Hospital in partnership with Dr. Atala's lab at Wake Forest.

Instead of waiting for a donated bladder, Katherine would grow a replacement.

Dr. Atala removed a small piece of Katherine's malfunctioning bladder and from it isolated about ten thousand adult stem cells, which he used as tiny tissue factories. Rather than leaving Katherine's bladder stem cells sleeping within a failing organ, Dr. Atala woke them up and set the factory machinery to work creating new bladder tissue, and lots of it.

He'd spent fifteen years perfecting the technique. You see, growing tissue isn't as easy as putting a sample in a petri dish and sticking it in an incubator. Each tissue type in the human body needs a specific blend of amino acids, electrolytes, sugars, and other factors to live and grow—the body is like a car with hundreds of microclimate controls, each designed for the purpose of providing the tissue with the fickle climate it needs. For fifteen years, Atala (and for one hundred years, doctors before him) had worked through educated guess, trial, error, and revision to perfect the right nutrient-protein shake for bladder tissue.

But even with healthy bladder tissue in a dish, a flat cell mat may make a good patch, but it can't take the place of an organ. And so Atala's lab led the way in engineering another kind of petri dish. Once Katherine's stem cells had been harvested and concentrated, Atala seeded them onto a 3D model that would replace her bladder. The model was made of collagen, the fibrous protein that connects and supports skin, bone, and muscle. This scaffold would be implanted with the stem cells grown around it and would then simply biodegrade over time. The replacement for Katherine's bladder started to grow, from the original ten thousand stem cells to more than 1.5 billion cells, which crept around the 3D model like hands cupping a cricket.

In a couple of weeks, Dr. Atala had a perfect replacement sitting in a dish in a lab at Wake Forest. Not only that, but it was Katherine's perfect replacement—one that had never been inside her body but built from her own cells nonetheless. And so when surgeons removed Katherine's hardened, dying organ and replaced it with the supple new one, it was sleight-of-hand magic, with the doctors as magicians and Katherine's body as the wide-eyed audience—the doctors made the switch and the body barely noticed the difference. Unlike transplants with donated organs, there is little fear that a patient's body will reject tissue grown from its own stem cells.

A couple weeks later, the bladderlike tube had healed into Katherine's urinary system. She didn't have to wear a diaper, and the new, elastic bladder held the toxic liquid without returning it to her kidneys. A lifetime of dialysis? Gone. A lifetime of incontinence? Gone. The junior prom?

Yes. Four years later, Katherine wore a low-cut, champagne-colored dress.

Six other children ranging from toddlers to teens, and all with spina bifida, benefited from the same clinical trial of bladder replacement. Even at this early stage in the treatment's development, six more kids saw their futures go from shortened and restricted to their equivalents of low-cut, champagne-colored dresses. The treatment was a success in seven of seven cases.

According to the American Cancer Society, in 2012 an estimated 73,510 new cases of bladder cancer will be diagnosed in the United States and 14,880 people will die from the disease. Maybe you know a patient. Maybe you will next year. Maybe you are or will be one of them yourself. Now there's hope. Generating a replacement for a bladder using a patient's stem cells is quickly going from a one-of-a-kind study of seven children toward a standard treatment in a physician's bag of tricks.

Having broken through the barrier of the first stem-cell-grown replacement for an organ, Wake Forest didn't stop with bladders. For example, the university reported in March 2011 that in conjunction with the Metropolitan Autonomous University in Mexico City, it had moved downstream from the bladder to urinary tubes.

Like Katherine's case, in which the common procedure of bladder repair with intestinal tissue was an imperfect fix at best, the common procedure for replacing damaged urethras with tissue grafts from the lining of the cheek frequently leads to complications. "These grafts, which can have failure rates of more than 50 percent, often become narrowed, leading to infections, difficulty urinating, pain, and bleeding," said Atlantida-Raya Rivera, director of the Tissue Engineering Laboratory at the Hospital Infantil de México Federico Gómez (HIMFG), Wake Forest's partner in Mexico City.

The two institutions worked to make a better option. Their first patients were five boys, three of whom had widespread injuries due to pelvic trauma and two of whom had had previous failed urethra replacement surgeries. "When they first came in, they [each] had a leg bag that drains urine, and they have to carry this bag everywhere they go," Atala told National Public Radio. "It's uncomfortable and painful. So these children were mostly sitting or bed-bound."

Like Katherine's procedure, the doctors grew samples of these boys' own tissue around three-dimensional scaffolds—in this case, models of urethra tubes. Once cells had grown to cover the biodegradable scaffolds, doctors removed the boys' damaged urethras and sewed the new tubes into place, replacing the entire segment that runs from the prostate to the outside—considered the most difficult to repair.

Because the tissue was grown from patients' own cells, there was little chance of rejection. Once the cells were implanted, the boys' bodies nourished the growing cells as if these cells were the bodies' own—which, of course, they were—and in 2011, these five boys completed their six-year follow-up checks. As measured by lack of nighttime leaking, straining to urinate, and urinary tract infections, all five urethras were functioning perfectly.

"These findings suggest that engineered urethras can be used successfully in patients and may be an alternative to the current treatment, which has a high failure rate," said Atala.

Now surgeons are using these techniques to grow vascular tissue—blood vessels—from patients' stem cells. And because some stem cells can make many tissues, these seed cells used to make blood vessels needn't even be from exactly the tissue they're replacing. Stem cells found in bone marrow can become any type of tissue found in the skin/muscle/blood-vessel system. Removed from a patient's marrow and seeded on long, spaghettilike molds, these cells are coaxed into forming replacement arteries for people undergoing bypass surgery. And in some cases, injections of stem cells can help patients regrow arteries in their own bodies directly, using the body's own machinery to tell the cells what to become and where.

For example, in 2009, sixty-six-year-old Reginald Smith had lost the ability to walk because of the buildup of plaque clogging the arteries that supplied blood to his legs. "It felt like the muscles were going to break in half, it was so painful," Reginald told ABC News. In fact, similar peripheral artery disease affects 20 percent of Americans older than sixty-five and can lead to ulcers, to gangrene, and eventually to amputations. Doctors injected stem cells into thirty sites in Reginald's legs, and within three days the oxygen level in his leg muscles had jumped from a dismal 43 percent to a reasonable 67 percent. Simply, his body had used the stem cells to grow natural bypasses around the clogged arteries in his legs.

There's much, much more.

In 2008, tuberculosis infected the windpipe leading to the left lung of thirty-year-old Sophia Castiglio, leaving her unable to climb a flight of stairs or take care of her children. Sophia found herself constantly panting for breath, even when resting. Before stem cells, the only fix would have been a transplant (with a long, uncertain wait and a high chance of rejection) or removal of the infected windpipe and Sophia's left lung along with it. But in June 2008, British surgeons turned to tissue engineering with Sophia's own adult stem cells. First they harvested and concentrated these cells, and then they seeded them onto a scaffold made from a section of donated windpipe. The stem cells grew down around the scaffold, and surgeons switched the tubercular windpipe connecting Sophia's trachea to her left lung with the lab-grown artificial pipe.

"I was scared at the beginning because I was the first patient but had confidence and trusted the doctors," said Sophia. "I am now enjoying life and am very happy that my illness has been cured." Five months after the surgery, not only could she take care of her children, but when she could find a babysitter and time in her tight schedule, Sophia went dancing.

Since Sophia's success several other stem cell trachea implants have been done, including in a twelve-year-old Irish boy who was born with a congenital deformity of his windpipe.

In addition to the existing therapies of replacements for bladders, urethras, and blood vessels, on the horizon are replacements for livers and kidneys. Again at Wake Forest, researcher Pedro Baptista described a new twist when growing a replacement liver—instead of seeding stem cells onto a plastic scaffold, Baptista treated an existing animal liver to remove its cells, leaving only the structural, collagen architecture. Then he injected human liver stem cells into the architecture, where they grew, filling out the structure.

The livers Baptista made were small—only about an inch in diameter and weighing about 0.20 ounces—and the technology needed to grow livers to the pound or more needed by the human body is still a ways off. Still, even now these tiny, functional human livers can be used for other, important medical purposes, including evaluating the safety of new drugs. "This would more closely mimic drug metabolism in the human liver, something that can be difficult to reproduce in animal models," said Baptista.

Until then, companies like the biotechnology company StemCells are pioneering the use of, for example, human liver engrafting cells, to support struggling livers without the need to replace the entire organ. Dr. Maria Millan, head of the liver program at the company, tells the story of a baby she treated who was born with a metabolic enzyme defect that required an immediate liver transplant. "We saved her life," says Millan, "but I believe that we can and will come up with a better way to treat our patients—through cell therapy."

Toward this goal, Millan is working to create techniques to transplant stem cells rather than entire organs. The concentrated mixture of liver stem cells Millan and other StemCell scientists created, known as hLEC, shows both in lab and animal studies the ability to produce important proteins needed for proper metabolic function.

From livers to kidneys: with ninety thousand people on the nationwide kidney transplant waiting list, Wake Forest hopes to replace or repair renal tissue. Already, the university has grown functional kidney cells and placed them in a mechanical, kidney-like device that's proved effective in mice. But even away from growing a fully functional replacement organ, researchers are experimenting with using kidney stem cells to grow cells that can be injected directly into underperforming kidneys, in hopes of regenerating or renewing the organ without the need for replacement. The university writes, "We foresee a time when cell therapy will replace damaged kidney tissue. Preliminary studies show that the injected cells are able to form tubular structures and have some evidence that they are integrated into native tissue."

And what is a bunny without the ability to reproduce? In a tissue-engineering success story that will certainly be appreciated by female rabbits, Wake Forest used stem cells to successfully grow male rabbit erectile tissue (that's what we call inserting levity into a book of science). Known as the corpora cavernosa penis, two columns of this sponge-like tissue are bound together with connective tissue and covered with skin, and they fill with blood during an erection. After Wake Forest doctors used stem cells to grow the tissue and then implanted it in the underperforming male rabbits, the repaired animals had normal sexual function and produced offspring (as rabbits are wont to do). Functional testing of the implanted tissue showed that vessel pressure within the erectile tissue was normal, that blood flowed smoothly through it as early as one month after implantation, and that veins drained normally after erection.

"These results are encouraging," said Dr. Atala. "They indicate the possibility of using laboratory-engineered tissue in men with erectile dysfunction who require reconstructive procedures. A lack of erectile tissue currently prevents us from restoring sexual function to these patients."

In all, the body parts being explored for stem cell regeneration at Wake Forest include blood vessel, bone, cartilage, cornea, diaphragm, ear, heart, heart valve, intestine, nerve, neuron, ovary, pancreas, prostate, salivary gland, muscle, tendon, and uterus. Some of these replacement parts are ready for installation. Ideally, others will be soon.

But recently, University of Missouri physicist Gabor Forgacs designed a sci-fi-sounding bio-printer that may speed some of Wake Forest's organ regeneration goals. The bio-printer works by spraying layers of stem cells, which stack into complex 3D shapes. Believe it or not, this is just a fancier version of the ink-jet printer most of us have attached to our computers. Instead of microscopic droplets of colored inks, the bio-printer squirts tiny droplets of nutrients containing stem cells.

"We need the ink; we call it the bio-ink. We need the paper; we call it the bio-paper. We need the printer, the bio-printer," says Forgacs. Basically, the printer draws stem cell shapes on sheets of bio-paper. Stacking these sheets, each with a slightly offset stem cell image, results in a paper tower and within it a tall 3D shape of stem cells. Then Forgacs's lab gives the stem cells in this shaped tower the cocktail they need to grow, and the developing cellular structure pushes through the bio-paper, fusing into the 3D printed shape.

Forgacs used his bio-printer to spray stem cells in the shape of a chicken heart. Like the collagen model of Katherine Manner's bladder, the bio-paper eventually biodegraded, leaving behind the exact 3D shape of a chicken heart. The muscle knew what to do: "We print the block of tissue and eventually would like that tissue to synchronously beat just as a heart would, and it does," said Forgacs. Supplied with nutrients and stimulated with the equivalent of a pacemaker, Forgacs's bio-printed chicken heart started to beat.

Forgacs hopes one day he will be able to bio-print not only hearts but livers and pancreases on demand, using the seeds of a patient's own stem cells. When that time comes, you will no longer need to check the organ donor box on your driver's license, simply because patients will be able to grow their own transplants. Forgacs hopes to develop a portable version of the bio-printer that battlefield medics could use to print layers of cells to treat deep wounds.

As for Katherine Manner, former president George W. Bush held a press conference with her, saying of her treatment, "Her doctors took a piece of her bladder, isolated the healthy stem cells, and used them to grow a new bladder in a laboratory—which they then transplanted into her. And here she stands, healthy."

At home in 2006, Katherine said to a CNN news crew, "I'm happy. I can run around and do a lot of things that I wasn't able to do because I was always afraid that I was going to have an accident or something. Now I can just go and go out with my friends. Go do whatever I want and not have to have worries about it." In 2010, Katherine graduated from Wesleyan University.

Today, medical science is reaching levels of knowledge that up to now only science fiction writers could imagine and make us dream about. Tomorrow it will be commonplace. For millions of Americans with organ disease or malfunction, there's more than new hope—there's treatment. And for kids like Katherine, there's a new normal that allows her to "go do whatever" without worries, which at the end of the day is what stem cell science is all about.

Chapter 2

Heart and Vascular Disease

"I had my first heart attack at thirty-nine, then the next one at forty. I had another one five years ago, and that was even after I had lost 135 pounds, was walking two miles a day, and going to the gym. I felt great and then *bang*," said Karen Parcher in an interview with the Texas Heart Institute. In her father's family, every one of three generations of males died of heart failure before age fifty. Still, even after three heart attacks, in 2006 Karen remained a workaholic—owner of her own event planning, cookie, and catering business in Montgomery, Alabama. She couldn't imagine slowing down.

Then *bang*. Again. Karen had a fourth heart attack. "After four heart attacks, I wondered what God had in store for me," she said. This time, restricted blood flow had killed enough heart muscle that doctors expected a fifth heart attack soon. Which one would be fatal? Doctors put her on the heart transplant waiting list, meaning that her condition had reached "end stage"—the point at which all other treatments had failed. While wait times on the list can vary, it was likely Karen would have to survive between six months and three years before a donor heart would become available, her heart weakening all the while. And even if she received a transplant, the ten-year heart transplant survival rate is only 50 percent.

But her mother had recently heard about another option. She wrote an impassioned letter to the Texas Heart Institute, which had just started a first-of-its-kind clinical trial exploring a stem cell treatment for end-stage heart disease. A month later, Karen brought cookies for the doctors in Houston who would evaluate her for the study. "I couldn't say two words without having to take a breath—I was always out of breath. I needed a wheelchair to get around the hospital for my tests," she said.

Thirty patients would be enrolled in the study, twenty of whom would get injections of stem cells straight into their hearts and ten of whom would receive a placebo.

Doctors at the Texas Heart Institute harvested Karen's bone marrow from her pelvis (hip bone). From this marrow, they concentrated stem cells marked with a protein called CD34. Cells with this protein on their outer cell wall are called CD34+ cells, and distilling these CD34+ cells from bone marrow results in a sort of stem cell slurry that the National Institutes of Health calls "a mixture of stem cells, progenitors, and white blood cells of varying degrees of maturity."

Researchers had shown in the lab that when this CD34+ mix comes in contact with heart tissue damaged by a heart attack, the stem cells promote the growth of new blood vessels needed to bring nutrients to damaged tissue and may excite growth factors in the damaged tissue that aid repair. It had worked in a petri dish, it had worked with mice, and now it was time to try the procedure with the first batch of humans, including Karen Parcher.

With twenty patients in the experimental stem cell group compared to ten in the control group, it would be a tense wait until Karen's six-month visit, when she would learn if she'd been injected with stem cells or with a placebo.

At about the same time, in Las Vegas, Donald Carlotti was waiting for his own heart transplant. At forty-nine years old, married with two young kids, in an interview with one of this book's authors, Dr. Max Gomez, Donald described his normal day: "On Wednesdays to Sunday I'd be up early in the morning to play with my little one because she gets me up at 5:30, quarter to six in the morning. Watch Nickelodeon or Noggin, whichever one, you know. And then I go to the casino, and I do my work."

After work, Donald said, he would usually "go home, have dinner, play with the kid, hang out, and then hop on the treadmill before I go to sleep."

What did he do between mornings and evenings spent playing with his three-year-old? Donald is a professional gambler, and his work is betting horses. "I play New York as my main track of the day. Belmont, Aqueduct—I play the Florida tracks, Santa Anita, California. I bet my horses—root, yell, scream, calm down after a race, and go on to the next one. I do pretty good," he says in an accent born of a childhood in Brooklyn and Queens.

But apparently the never-ending cycle of anticipation, stress, and release wasn't good for his heart, especially in combination with diabetes. In 2004, Donald got bronchitis and with it came a little shortness of breath. But even after a course of antibiotics and the recovery from other symptoms, his breath never came back. "I picked up my one-year-old, walked about eight feet, thought I ran like a twenty-six-mile marathon. Drove myself to the hospital, walked in, said I was having a heart attack."

After triage, it turned out that the cholesterol blockages in Donald's heart were so extensive that the angioplasty balloons couldn't push through. "They told me to bring my family in because blood flow was almost nothing and it didn't look good," he says. "I just said that I don't want to die right now. I have too much—I have kids and a wife. I can't die now." Donald went onto the heart transplant list, but his diabetes hurt his priority.

After a year of waiting, Donald's worried brother started to explore other options. He told Donald about an experimental (and unregulated) stem cell therapy in Thailand, and Donald packed his bags. But his brother kept calling around and eventually got in touch with an officer at the biotechnology company NeoStem.

The officer suggested that Donald see a doctor at the University of Pittsburgh who was enrolling patients in a new clinical trial that used stem cells as a healing agent after open-heart surgery. "It worked out even better," Donald says. "Who wants to go to Thailand when they can go to Pittsburgh? Shorter flight."

Who, indeed!

Donald went to Pittsburgh, and after tests, the doctor told him there was good news and bad news: "He said the blockages are really bad, and you're in bad shape. But the good news is I can fix you up—with stem cells and an open-heart surgery," Donald recalls.

So that was what they did.

And at this same time, while Karen Parcher was waiting to hear the results of her clinical trial and Donald Carlotti was on the operating table, Bernie van Zyl was waiting to die of congestive heart failure. A retired engineer and researcher, just before Christmas 2000 Bernie had started feeling congestion in his chest, and so he scheduled an exam for December 18. On December 17, he felt worse and drove himself to a walk-in clinic, imagining he had a cold or maybe walking pneumonia. The doctor at the clinic agreed that a cold was likely and sent Bernie home with suggestions for over-the-counter medicines. That evening, after taking his cold medicines, Bernie lay down.

"Suddenly, I felt a terrible pain in the center of my chest," he says. "It was as if someone had hit me with an axe." His wife, Lynn, drove him half a block to the hospital that was at the end of their street.

Bernie died in the emergency room—his heart stopped.

And then he woke up. He recalls, "A doctor looking closely into my eyes said, 'Your heart stopped, but we managed to get it started again. How do you feel?'"

Doctors call this type of sudden heart attack a "widow maker"—only 10 percent of patients whose hearts stop in the emergency room ever get it started again. Bernie later described being a bit disappointed that he hadn't seen a white light. His heart stopped again, and doctors had to shock it back into action for a second time while Bernie was undergoing bypass surgery for a completely blocked left main heart artery. After the surgery, his heart again refused to beat on its own, so doctors hooked him to a heart-lung machine that did his breathing and beating for him. His family arrived to say their good-byes.

Eventually, against the odds, Bernie's heart started beating on its own, and eventually, gingerly, doctors removed him from the heart-lung machine. When his wife went home that evening, there was a message on their answering machine reminding them of the heart stress test that Bernie had scheduled for the next day—the one that would almost certainly have shown the blockage.

At the hospital, Bernie refused to sleep, imagining that every time he drifted off, it would be his last descent into cardiac arrest. Finally, doctors had to call his wife back to the hospital, where she pulled a recliner close to her husband's bed. They slept that way, with her arm snaked through IV tubes and monitoring wires and across Bernie's chest.

A month later, Bernie left the hospital, but his prognosis was still bad. Donor hearts are few and precious; the horrible truth is that they're generally reserved for patients in whom they will do the most good. Older patients may not have the overall strength to thrive after a transplant, and the years of quality life gained in older patients tends to be fewer than in younger patients. Traditionally, age fifty-five was seen as the upper limit for heart transplants, but with life expectancy increasing and with surgical advances, this upper transplant age has generally been pushed to sixty-five, and some places, such as Jackson Memorial Hospital in Miami, Florida, even transplant at age seventy. According to *Transplant Living*, in 2011 the average cost of a heart transplant approached $1 million and a lifetime to follow of expensive immunosuppressive drugs to prevent rejection of a new heart. Still, Bernie wasn't eligible for a transplant, as he was deemed "too well" to be put on the list.

Bernie lived for five years, always on the cusp, fearful to sleep in case he never woke up. "I'm probably the most optimistic person in the world," he says, "and I knew I would find something. But at that point, it was hard doing research, because I was awake maybe four hours a day. The rest of the time I was in bed asleep. And I really had to push myself to do the work." Finally, after five years, he found what he was looking for—a clinical trial in Boston. It was very much like Karen Parcher's trial at the Texas Heart Institute, in which doctors would inject Bernie with the drug Neupogen (granulocyte colony-stimulating factor) to encourage his bone marrow to release CD34+ stem cells into his blood, where they could be easily harvested and injected near his damaged heart tissues.

But despite the seeming similarities of Karen Parcher, Donald Carlotti, and Bernie van Zyl, these are three distinct cases, each with its own fascinating results.

At her six-month visit, doctors handed Karen a small white

envelope that would tell her whether she had received stem cells or the placebo. "My hands were shaking like a leaf," she recalls. "I pulled out the paper, and there were two little words: stem cells!" These cells that had been harvested from Karen's hip and then concentrated in the lab had helped heal her heart. Current science still doesn't know exactly how or why, but it appears that instead of spitting out cells that become new heart tissue, these CD34+ stem cells may have acted like a biological cheering squad, promoting the growth of new blood vessels (angiogenesis), decreasing swelling, and potentially exciting growth factors in tissue that was previously at death's door—in other words, acting like a cellular Advil and helping this damaged tissue repair itself. Or perhaps these CD34+ cells stimulated the stem cells that had been lying dormant in Karen's heart, waiting for a wake-up call. (More on these "native" stem cells hiding in most or all of our organs and tissues later.)

A 2006 Harvard study published in the journal *Molecular Therapy* described the results this way: "[CD34+ stem cells] . . . restored early cardiac function . . . despite transient engraftment [and] low levels of . . . differentiation . . . Early paracrine [repair] mechanisms mediated by MSC [mesenchymal stem cells] are responsible for enhancing the survival of existing myocytes and . . . could alter the secretion of various cytokines and growth factors." In English, this basically confirms that stem cells can encourage damaged tissue to grow, thus repairing hearts without themselves becoming heart cells.

Whatever the case, the injection of stem cells into Karen's heart made a drastic difference in her life and allowed her to resume her regular activity at her catering business. "I was in the 'waiting to die' stage when I was introduced to the Texas Heart Institute," says Karen. "Now I can walk three blocks without getting winded. I think it's a miracle. I feel so blessed."

Today, an important refinement makes Karen's treatment even better. The biotechnology company Amorcyte, a subsidiary of NeoStem, is developing a therapy that uses a technique to harvest CD34+ stem cells without the use of Neupogen. If you remember, this is the drug that encouraged Karen's bone marrow to release CD34+ cells into her bloodstream—but in addition to pulling them from where they "should be" in the bone marrow, Neupogen also dumbs down the ability of these stem cells to naturally migrate to damaged areas. Instead, harvested without Neupogen, the CD34+ stem cells can be injected not invasively into the heart but simply into the artery that was blocked, where they then migrate (along the SDF1 gradient) on their own to the areas in need of repair. This increases blood flow to the dead, ischemic tissue and supports the surrounding healthy tissue that, due to the heart attack, must work harder to compensate.

For example, in an interview with one of this book's authors, Mack Roberts described a heart attack in 2007 that felt like "somebody had taken a pickax and repeatedly hit me between the shoulder blades in the back." After being stabilized at a hospital in Gainesville, Florida, Mack was transported to Emory University, where Dr. Arshed Quyyumi treated him as part of an ongoing clinical trial of Amorcyte's stem cell product AMR–001, which is a concentrated mixture of a patient's own CD34+ stem cells. In 2011, Mack said, "I really don't think I have any ill effects from the heart attack. I feel fine. I still go out and do things I need to do. We've got ten acres of property and we have some rental cabins on it. There's always something to do. I'll cut a tree down. I'll haul a tree out of the woods. I'll do a lot of different things."

The thirty-one-person Amorcyte AMR–001 trial (CD34CXCR4) showed that patients who were treated with 10 million or more of a specific population of their own stem cells had an increase of oxygenated blood through new blood vessel formation feeding the damaged and surrounding heart muscle than did patients treated with fewer or no stem cells. The results were so promising that the Food and Drug Administration (FDA) has given the green light for a 160-person, phase II clinical trial using AMR–001, which is now well under way.

As for Donald Carlotti, his stem cells were used in a slightly different way—to promote healing after open-heart surgery. Donald remembers lying in the recovery room, looking up at his wife and his one-year-old, whom his wife had to smuggle past the nurses. "I just started looking around the room, and something in my own brain said I just can't die now, just not time to go," Donald says.

As heart patients know, the term *ejection fraction* refers to the percentage of blood that is pumped out of the right and left ventricles with each heartbeat. A high percent is good—it means your heart is efficiently moving blood through itself and thus through the rest of your body. A normal ejection fraction is 58 percent, and an article on the Cleveland Clinic's website says that below 35 percent, a patient "may be at risk of life-threatening irregular heartbeats." Before Donald's surgery and recovery, his ejection fraction was 13 percent—only about an eighth of the blood contained in his heart was being pumped out with each beat. By his six-month visit, it had increased to 47 percent.

"I played ball my whole life," says Donald. "I mean I played in New York on every flag football league, softball league, all over the place. Three months after surgery, I've been playing ball, you know, just going to the gym running around, doing what I have to do. I feel great." The results of his clinical trial were eventually published in the journal *Nature*.

"Where I was at September '04 and where I am now in January '07—never thought I could be in this position," Donald told Dr. Max. "I think I'll be around for a while, which mentally makes me feel good. I'll watch my kids grow up, and this fear I had a couple of years ago is that if I pass away now, will my one-year-old remember me? Will she know who I am or who I was? I mean, I walk as fast as people run normally . . . I thought it would slow me down, but it really didn't."

Bernie van Zyl's results are a little less straightforward, but even with their twist, they provide compelling evidence of the power of stem cells to heal the heart.

Like Karen Parcher, before drawing blood and concentrating stem cells from it, Dr. Douglas Losordo gave Bernie the drug Neupogen, which (again) encouraged his bone marrow to release more CD34+ stem cells into his bloodstream. Then, after an easy blood draw, doctors had a fairly stem-cell-rich blood mixture, which they further concentrated in the lab. "They assigned me a number, and I became number 19 in the study. And the only person who knew who got the real stem cells was a technician who bagged them and put a number on them," Bernie says.

For five months, Bernie felt as if he'd gotten the placebo. "I was still being wheeled through the airports in a wheelchair and things like that," he says. Then at the end of the fifth month, he started feeling much better. This good health lasted for a month and then—poof!—it was gone. "I lost my strength, lost my stamina. I was back exactly where I had started from," Bernie recalls. From nothing to everything and then back to nothing. What had happened? Being a scientist himself, Bernie hypothesized that perhaps the stem cell treatment took time to kick in and then offered a fleeting window of effectiveness before being overrun by his condition and eventually proving unsuccessful.

The doctor in charge of the trial petitioned the FDA to "unblind" the study, and when they did, Bernie learned that he had been given the placebo. Instead of being injected with his own stem cells, he had been injected with saline solution.

"So the question is, why did I feel better?" Bernie asks. "A placebo effect should have taken place much earlier. I should have said after a week or so, 'Oh gosh, I feel like a new person.' But that wasn't the case; it took five months."

It turns out the likely cause of Bernie's fleeting cure was the fact that even using Neupogen to encourage CD34+ stem cells to leave their caves in the bone marrow and circulate freely through the blood may have helped his heart. In fact, this increase in blood-borne stem cells pumping through the heart seems to take about five months to show health effects. But it's a temporary fix. "You don't get enough of them into your heart muscle. And so the repair is not sustained," Bernie says.

So, despite being in the placebo wing of the trial, Bernie experienced the health benefits of treatment with his own stem cells, however short-lived.

After learning he'd been given the placebo, Bernie had the option to undergo the real stem cell treatment. He did. "They put a catheter into the femoral artery in my leg, threaded the catheter into my heart, and then did a fairly remarkable thing—they mapped the inside of my heart, and they were able to define a line between where the heart muscle was good and where it had been damaged. They injected the stem cells at ten places along that dividing line," Bernie explains.

His health followed the same pattern it had after he'd been given the placebo. For five months, Bernie felt awful. And then five months after his stem cell treatment, he started to get back his stamina, and this time he kept it.

"Before I got the stem cell therapy, I had no energy whatsoever," he says. "As I mentioned, I slept most of the day because I didn't have the stamina or energy to do anything else. And now I work out on my exercise bike. I work out on a Nautilus. I swim, I walk, I don't know of any limitations whatsoever."

Bernie van Zyl wrote a book describing his experience, titled *How Adult Stem Cell Therapies Saved My Life*. On the cover, he holds a tennis racket.

In the twenty-four-person trial, the eighteen people who received stem cell injections all showed lasting improvements. Like Bernie, the six who were given the placebo all improved and then relapsed. When these six were then treated with CD34+ stem cells harvested from their blood, all six improved. In other words, when given the real treatment, all twenty-four people in this early study benefited from this rudimentary stem cell therapy.

"After your doctor says, 'I'm sorry, but there's nothing we can do for you, we've tried everything, perhaps you should get your affairs in order,' most people give up because they believe their doctor knows everything," says Bernie. "But in many cases he or she doesn't. My message to patients is take charge of your own case and don't give up."

Karen Parcher, Donald Carlotti, Mack Roberts, and Bernie van Zyl are four very different cardiac cases who underwent four different stem cell treatments. All of them are success stories.

With clinical trials run by Harvard, Emory, the Mayo Clinic, the University of Pittsburgh, and the Texas Heart Institute, and results published in such top scientific journals as *Nature*, the *New England Journal of Medicine*, and *Circulation*, the clinical journal of the American Heart Association, the application of adult stem cells harvested from a patient's blood and returned to their heart is one case in which stem cell treatments are more than a futurist's pipe dream—they're a pragmatist's go-to treatment.

If you want to get scientific, the abstract of a 2004 study published in the journal *Lancet* says it all: "Intracoronary transfer of autologous bone-marrow-cells promotes improvement of left-ventricular systolic function in patients after acute myocardial infarction."

This stem cell treatment is here today, now, saving lives. To add your name to the list with Karen, Mack, Donald, and Bernie, refer to this book's final chapter on how to find similar clinical trials.

While stem cell healing now seems to depend mostly on the ability of stem cells to kick-start damaged tissue by stimulating the creation of blood vessels (angiogenesis) and exciting growth factors, researchers are getting closer to tapping their full potential to generate completely new heart tissue. For example, a 2009 article in the *Journal of the American College of Cardiology* showed that CD34+ cells are not the only stem-like cells that mobilize into the bloodstream after a heart attack. Along with these cells is a fivefold increase in the number of circulating VSELs—the promising very small embryonic-like cells that live in the adult body but retain their pluripotency. In addition to promoting repair, these cells have the potential to become new heart tissue, as was shown in a phase I study conducted by Dr. Roberto Bolli and colleagues and published in the November 26, 2011, issue of the *Lancet*.

The future holds promise for heart patients with valve disease, too. Back at the Wake Forest lab of Anthony Atala, scientists are working to engineer entirely new heart valves. By starting with the valve from a pig heart, stripping away its cells, injecting the remaining collagen matrix with stem cells from a patient's blood, and exercising the new valve in a bioreactor engineered for the purpose, Atala has shown initial success in manufacturing new valves that match a patient's tissue. Like

Wake Forest's successes in transplanting lab-grown replacements for bladders, urethras, and blood vessels (described in chapter 1), it's only a matter of time before this novel heart valve makes its way into humans.

Also in 2009, a team at the University of Wisconsin–Madison showed that induced pluripotent stem cells—skin cells that had been reprogrammed back to their embryonic-like state—could be coaxed into creating beating heart cells in the lab. The university's news release states, "The discovery suggests that a patient's own skin cells could someday be used to repair damaged heart tissue."

Vascular insufficiency doesn't only affect the heart, which is why these technologies can't come soon enough for Jenny O'Reilly. On March 10, 2011, she told her story to a group of doctors and researchers from the California Institute for Regenerative Medicine (CIRM), a statewide organization created in 2004 by California Proposition 71, which raised $3 billion to fund stem cell research in California's universities and research institutions.

Since 1972, Jenny was a hairdresser who worked many hours on her feet and was wondering why her legs felt like tree trunks. She had battled peripheral artery disease, in which obstructions in the blood vessels of her legs and arms kept her tissues from getting the oxygen and nutrients they need to survive. According to the American Heart Association, peripheral artery disease affects about eight million Americans and increases a patient's risk of stroke and heart attack by four or five times. Tissue with reduced oxygen is also ripe for infections and gangrene.

"I had ulcers on my hands, my feet," says Jenny. "I'd get 'em filled up eventually. And then I had a toe that wouldn't heal." She went to her podiatrist, who gave her antibiotics, but without proper blood flow, the toe remained an open ulcer. Eventually she went to a vascular surgeon, but he didn't work below the ankle.

In 2004, Jenny started seeing Dr. John Laird, now director of the Vascular Center at the University of California, Davis. Dr. Laird immediately performed surgery to open three blockages in the arteries of Jenny's left leg. For four years, she returned two or three times a year to have her arteries scraped open. But in 2008, after she had the procedure again, the outcome was different. "By the time I was back in my room for recovery," she recalls, "my foot was cold. It ended up it was blocked up again."

Jenny lost her left leg below the knee. Dr. Laird suggested she explore stem cell therapies in hopes of saving her right. "If the stem cell research can encourage the arteries to rebuild, just think: I won't lose my right leg," Jenny says.

Could stem cells injected into Jenny's right leg encourage her body to grow new arteries, providing new pathways for blood to reach the decaying tissues of her feet? It's a compelling idea, and in fact is one that's already been tested.

On November 14, 2011, the biotechnology company Aastrom Biosciences reported the twelve-month follow-up results of its phase II clinical trial called RESTORE-CLI. The trial treated patients who had inadequate blood supply to their limbs (that is, critical limb ischemia) with a mixture of their own stem cells injected into twenty points in a dying lower thigh, calf, and foot. For a year after treatment, the team watched seventy-two patients for further tissue death and gangrene. The patients treated with the stem cell mixture called ixmyelocel-T showed a 62 percent reduction in these complications compared to patients treated with a placebo.

Now the RESTORE-CLI trial moves to phase III, the pivotal hurdle before potential approval by the FDA.

Jenny O'Reilly will undergo a similar procedure at UC Davis, and soon we'll know if stem cells succeed where near-constant artery scraping failed.

The United States isn't the only place where this technology is pushing forward. In Italy, Dr. Eugenio Caradonna is exploring similar uses of stem cells for peripheral artery disease and critical limb ischemia.

Does Dr. Caradonna's name ring a bell? Keep reading and it might. In St. Peter's Square in Vatican City on May 13, 1981, Mehmet Ali Agca fired four shots at Pope John Paul II. Two bullets lodged in the Pope's lower intestine, and two more hit his left hand and right arm. He was rushed to the Agostino Gemelli University Polyclinic where, in the course of a five-hour surgery, Pope John Paul II lost nearly three-quarters of his blood. The attending physician that day was Eugenio Caradonna.

In August 2011, Caradonna and colleagues from the John Paul II Catholic University of Campobasso, Italy, published the results of their own stem cell trial for critical limb ischemia in the respected journal *Vascular and Endovascular Surgery*. The subjects for this study were ten patients with critical limb ischemia who hadn't responded to traditional treatments and whose lack of circulation had left them looking at amputation as their next step. First, as with Bernie van Zyl, the Italian doctors treated these ischemia patients with a drug that encourages bone marrow to release stem cells into the bloodstream. Then doctors used a cutting-edge blood drawing and stem cell concentrating system developed by Harvest Technologies, which allowed them to develop the treatment's stem cell cocktail right at each patient's bedside within fifteen minutes. In the same operating room session, they then injected patients' concentrated mesenchymal stem cells into muscles surrounding the critical zones of ischemia. (Though the name sounds fancy, these "critical zones of ischemia" are generally easy to spot in these patients—they're the ones that are gray, soon to be black.)

Without this stem cell treatment, every one of these patients would have gone immediately to the operating room for amputation. In these ten Italian patients, seven avoided amputation of any kind, and three required amputation only of tissues far below the injected areas that had already decayed beyond repair.

The Italian team led by Dr. Caradonna went ten-for-ten in their first clinical trial of stem cells for critical limb ischemia. How many NBA basketball players can hit ten free throws in a row? The doctors write that after stem cell treatment, all ten patients showed the formation of new blood vessels in their ischemic limbs. In the "before" and "after" figures that illustrate their paper (available with a quick online search), blood vessels in the leg of one patient are seen in the "before" picture as a few small squiggles, like a Japanese ink drawing of a dying tree painted with watery ink. In the "after" picture, this tree has new branches, and the branches are confident and dark, filled with blood. Even to the untrained eye, it's obvious what has happened: the leg has grown new vessels.

Before stem cell therapies, patients like high-roller Donald Carlotti, busy Karen Parcher, and retired physicist Bernie van Zyl would have died of their diseases. Now they lived through them. And in Italy, ten patients who would have lost their legs kept them. This is the promise of stem cell research.

Chapter 3

Burns

In *Star Trek IV: The Voyage Home*, Dr. McCoy travels back in time to visit a hospital in the 1980s. Passing a woman on a gurney, groaning in the hallway, McCoy asks what's wrong, and the elderly patient croaks, "Dialysis!" McCoy responds, "What is this, the Dark Ages?" and hands her a pill. Later, the patient has grown a fully functional kidney. And as a standard tool in his medical kit, McCoy carries a gun that sprays new skin over the wounds and burns of Starship *Enterprise* crew members.

Of course, this is science fiction, not science fact. But stem cells can help us reach *Star Trek* creator Gene Roddenberry's vision. We've already seen the techniques of Anthony Atala at Wake Forest University to grow replacements for malfunctioning organs, and now there exists a fully functional spray gun that can coat ulcers and burns with a fine layer of stem cells that heal severe burns and other skin defects in days, not weeks.

It's a good thing—the standard treatment for large burns isn't pretty. Generally, surgeons start by removing any dead tissue, either slicing it away or, in a cutting-edge treatment that seems to support Dr. McCoy's accusations of modern medicine being no better than the Dark Ages, doctors can use a species of live maggots to eat away the necrotic skin. Really—in January 2004, the FDA granted permission to produce and sell maggots for use in cleaning dead tissue, or in some cases bacteria, from human wounds. In 2006, the procedure was used about fifty thousand times.

As bizarrely appealing as this is, it's only half the procedure. After a burn wound is cleaned, doctors generally cut healthy skin from an uninjured part of the body and graft it over the burned area. This creates double the area that requires healing, and in patients with burns over a large percentage of their body, it may have to be accomplished in stages over months, or grafting may have to be done with the skin of a cadaver when there's not enough unburned skin to use as a donor site. Existing synthetic skins are far from perfect, and techniques to grow a small sample of a patient's skin into a large patch needed for grafting take weeks or even months.

The skin is the body's biggest organ, and doctors and scientists are working toward being able to engineer replacement skin in the lab that would serve as a living biological dressing. According to an article on the Wake Forest Institute for Regenerative Medicine's website, this new skin "can act as a barrier and integrate into the patient's existing skin tissue, while at the same time reducing scarring and contraction."

Generally, this biological Band-Aid works by seeding skin stem cells onto sheets of biological material. The institute imagines storing these sheets of engineered skin in a national tissue bank, ready for immediate use. Other laboratories, such as the one run by Dr. Vincent Falanga at the Boston University School of Medicine, are working on a fibrin and stem cell mixture that can be applied in three treatments to a burn or nonhealing wound to get closure. In order to accelerate this promising approach to rapid wound healing, the US Department of Defense has funded further research being conducted by such companies as NeoStem.

Imagine the difference this could make to the 10 percent of all war casualties that are due to burns, or to the 1,103,300 firefighters in the United States (as of 2010, according to the National Fire Protection Association), more than 3,000 of whom were burned in 2010.

Unfortunately, replacement skin is also needed in times of mass casualties. And it was one of these mass-casualty situations in which a different skin regeneration technique saw its first big test.

On October 12, 2002, a suicide bomber detonated a backpack inside Paddy's Pub, a crowded and popular nightclub in the tourist district of Kuta on the Indonesian island of Bali. Twenty seconds later, another bomb in a white Mitsubishi van exploded across the street, leaving a three-foot crater in the ground. Paddy's Pub was leveled, and windows three blocks away in this dense residential and commercial district imploded from the force of the powerful car bomb. But the damage wasn't limited to the bomb's percussion. The terrorists had made the 2,250-pound van-bomb from a mixture of potassium chlorate, aluminum powder, sulfur, and TNT, connected by almost 500 feet of detonating cord. This combination made the explosion "thermobaric," meaning that in addition to the punch, it packed heat. As much as a bomb, this was a fire weapon, and the injuries it produced were mostly burns.

More than five hundred people were burned, most of them Australians in their twenties and thirties who were vacationing in Bali. One of them was Grigori Venadich, a twenty-six-year-old crane operator from the Sydney suburb of Coogee who was at Paddy's Pub on the first night of a Bali vacation that he hoped would help him get over the recent death of his father. The bomb pinned Grigori under burning timbers, and yet somehow amid the smoke, pain, and confusion, he managed to wrench himself free and crawl outside.

"That was divine intervention," Grigori told Perth's *Age* newspaper. "How I managed to get up and walk out of that bar, I just don't know." Burns covered 64 percent of his body.

Despite heroic actions by doctors and a handful of medically trained visitors who sprung into action, local hospitals were overwhelmed. Some victims were placed in hotel pools to ease the pain of their burns. Grigori and other more severe cases were flown to Australia for specialized treatment.

In the early morning hours of October 13, an airplane landed in Perth, and twenty-eight victims with burns covering between 2 and 92 percent of their bodies were rushed to the Royal Perth Hospital in Western Australia. Even in Perth, there weren't enough surgeons, wasn't enough cadaver skin to coat patients' burns, and on Grigori and other severe cases, there wasn't enough skin remaining to perform traditional grafts by transferring skin from elsewhere on their bodies.

Instead, Dr. Fiona Wood, head of the Royal Perth Hospital Burns Unit, mother of six, and daughter of a Yorkshire coal miner, reached for her device—a spray-on skin gun she had spent ten years developing.

From Grigori and the others, Wood harvested a postage-stamp-sized patch of skin, only about five one-thousandths of an inch deep. Working quickly, Wood and her staff used the enzyme trypsin to dissolve the structural material that held skin stem cells trapped in this tissue. And then, having mobilized the stem cells, Wood and her colleagues combined the patients' stem cells with a mixture of nutrients and growth factors and sprayed the stem-cell-rich cocktail onto their red and blistered burn areas. The stem cells from this postage stamp of skin were enough to seed a burned area the size of a sheet of paper.

The stem cells in this mixture quickly got to work generating new tissue. In less than a week, areas coated with this spray-on skin had healed, covered with new, elastic, scar-free skin that matched the patients' own—and with no risk of rejection associated with cadaver grafts or those grown from donors. Many of these horribly burned patients walked out of the hospital within the week, with drastically reduced scarring.

Grigori Venadich was not one of them. He lapsed into a coma.

"I hear the stories; I know what they're going through," Dr. Wood told the Australian Broadcasting Corporation. "I can feel their anguish. The mother who says, 'My husband died six weeks ago; this is my only son.' You can't be unaffected by that."

In all, 202 people died in the 2002 Bali bombings—88 Australians, 38 Indonesians, 24 from the United Kingdom, and the rest from countries ranging from the United States to South Africa to Taiwan. Without Fiona Wood's stem cell treatment, Grigori would almost certainly have been number 203. Instead, forty-four days later, Grigori woke from his coma. Not long after, he limped from the hospital.

"It feels fantastic; words can't describe it," he told the *Age*. Grigori's case is an example of the combined power of God and science—what he called "divine intervention," which guided his escape from the burning rubble, paired with Dr. Wood's stem cell treatment. These forces in tandem allowed him to walk out of the Royal Perth Hospital on January 7, 2003, with one crutch. A picture of Grigori leaving the hospital shows him smiling, flanked by family and friends, and with the only visible sign of his burns being minor discoloration to the skin of his forehead and one side of his face.

Since 2002, Wood's stem cell spray gun has been in wide use in Australia. It's proved especially useful in pediatric burn cases, where skin grafts or letting the burn heal with scar tissue frequently results in tissue that doesn't grow with the patient, necessitating a series of surgeries to stretch the healed skin—scar tissue, really—to fit the growing child.

Take the case of a boy named Joe, who at twelve months old pulled a cup of scalding hot tea onto himself, completely covering his chest, left arm, and neck. Pictures on the website of the biotechnology company Avita Medical are graphic, showing Joe's bright red burned chest, which could be the picture of a wet red balloon. Doctors knew that over the next eighteen years, Joe would more than triple his size but that grafts or scar tissue would not, so instead of these traditional treatments, they reached for Fiona Wood's spray-on stem cell gun.

Six days later, Joe left the hospital.

During a follow-up visit twenty-one months later, doctors snapped a picture of Joe, who was now almost three years old. In this follow-up photo, the red balloon of his chest is replaced by a picture with absolutely no visible trace of scarring or injury of any kind. Rather than an injury that could easily have defined his life, Joe looks like a typical, rough-and-ready little boy. The medical check confirmed no evidence of wound breakdown or thick scarring.

Doctors used the same treatment with six-year-old Karl, whose spina bifida left him with no feeling in his feet and so no clue that the summer sand he was standing on was melting off the sole of his left foot. Doctors harvested a postage-stamp-size bit of skin from Karl's bottom and fifteen minutes later sprayed the stem cell mixture onto Karl's horrifically burned foot. Seven days after treatment Karl was released from the hospital. If you were to look at the photo taken at his six-month follow-up visit, you'd be hard-pressed to tell the difference between the soles of his left and right feet.

Again, imagine this treatment for firefighters or for soldiers injured in combat. In fact, you can do more than imagine it. In 2009, Wood's ReCell technology, which had previously been approved for use in Canada, Mexico, Europe, and many other countries, came to the United States in the form of a clinical trial cosponsored by the Armed Forces Institute of Regenerative Medicine, the University of Pittsburgh, and Wake Forest University.

Jonathan Ache, a thirty-something state police officer from Pennsylvania, was one of the first patients treated. He told his story to a news team from National Geographic Channel. "I attended a Fifth of July party at a friend's house. I was standing next to the bonfire, and an individual decided to throw a cup of gasoline on the fire."

The fire roared, and Jonathan turned his right side toward the flames while staggering backward. "The worst part was the whole right side of my face here, my ear, my neck, and my shoulder, and the entire top part of my arm," he told the National Geographic team, pointing to the areas that were burned. In all, he suffered second-degree burns over a huge area of his upper right side.

"The arm kind of looked like a piece of charred meat, like a hot dog that was left on a grill too long," Jonathan said. When he arrived at the emergency room, the skin of his right upper arm and shoulder was sloughing off like the ripples of a soft-serve cone left too long in the sun.

Dr. Jörg Gerlach of the University of Pittsburgh's McGowan Institute for Regenerative Medicine describes how he and his team treated Jonathan. "Skin cell spraying is like paint spraying," Gerlach says. "It takes like one and a half hours. To take the biopsy, to isolate the cells, and to spray the cells."

In the film (titled *The Skin Gun*; watch the trailer at chan nel.nationalgeographic.com), Jonathan describes the results of this simple ninety-minute procedure. "They did it on a Friday and my follow-up was that Monday, and the burn unit said it was healed, completely healed," he says.

In the National Geographic video, the camera starts wide on Jonathan, who stands with his shirt off at forty-five degrees to the camera, showing his burned right side. He looks fit and comfortable. Then the camera zooms in on his burned shoulder. Only, you can't tell it was ever burned. The skin has healed so completely that it's maybe just a shade pinker than the undamaged skin of his back. In comparison to the skin newly grown with a mixture of his own stem cells, his natural skin looks old.

If patients continue to show results even half as successful as those of Jonathan, the way spray-on skin tests throughout the world have, bedside kits that allow harvesting, mixing, and spraying stem cells on burn areas will be available in the United States by 2013.

In Jonathan Ache's case, this spray-on skin allows a Fifth of July bonfire mistake to be an infrequent bad memory instead of an everyday reminder. After the Bali bombings, divine intervention saved Grigori Venadich, and spray-on skin healed him. And in the case of little Joe who burned himself with a cup of tea, this spray-on skin turned an injured little boy back into simply a little boy.

In all these cases, stem cell medicine not only healed wounds but changed lives. And Jonathan, Grigori, and little Joe are the first faces of a technology that will affect millions.

Chapter 4

Brain Trauma and Stroke

In a February 2011 ABC News video, Jackson Dwyer's father put a finger by the twelve-year-old's left eye and another on the back of Jackson's head. "This is where his head hit the car in the accident," Jackson's father said. Then he held his fingers about a softball's-width apart and put them above Jackson's left eyebrow, saying, "And that section right there was actually crushed into multiple pieces."

The accident was in 2009, a head-on car crash in Texas. Jackson was cut from the car and rushed to the hospital, where surgeons diagnosed him with a massive concussion and a stroke. "I remember waking up and wondering why I couldn't move the left side of my body," Jackson told ABC. The surgeons told his parents to expect brain damage.

According to a study by the Mayo Clinic published in the *Journal of Insurance Medicine*, stroke caused by a burst blood vessel kills half its victims; among the survivors, a third lose the ability to care for themselves, and three-quarters lose the ability to perform at least some of the tasks of daily living.

But it happened that Memorial Hermann Hospital, where Jackson was taken (also the hospital where Congresswoman

Gabrielle Giffords rehabbed after being shot in the head), was enrolling patients in an early clinical trial that involved harvesting patients' mesenchymal stem cells and injecting them into damaged areas of the brain. Jackson's parents signed the forms, and the results were dramatic. Not only did Jackson regain movement on the left side of his body, he actually walked out of the hospital eight days later with no apparent brain damage. He played baseball and made the honor roll that year. In the fall of 2011, an Internet search for *Jackson Dwyer* first turns up a couple stories about his brain injury and treatment but are quickly followed by his results from tennis tournaments.

Near the end of the ABC interview, his father said, "We do feel incredibly lucky that not only can we hug him but he can hug us back."

Of the ten kids in this University of Texas study performed at Memorial Hermann, almost all of them benefited from the procedure.

How is this possible?

Well, the brain is tricky. Once a human reaches adulthood, stem cells remain active in only two areas of the brain, continuing to make an appreciable number of new neurons. Your hippocampus is responsible for packaging new memories for storage deeper in the brain—its stem cells stay active. And your brain's olfactory bulb—responsible for detecting smells—does the same.

Everywhere else in the brain, neurons that die aren't replaced. This is one thing that makes brain injury so insidious. Unlike Mary Shelley's famous monster, once a neuron dies, you can't shock, prod, or engineer it back to life. A dead neuron is irreplaceable except in the hippocampus and olfactory bulb, where new neurons are born to take dead neurons' place.

So, what happened to Jackson Dwyer that day in 2009 in an operating room in Texas?

The California Institute for Regenerative Medicine (CIRM) suggests a possible answer. "Stem cells at first seemed ideal replacement parts, living Legos for stroke-damaged brains," said an article in CIRM's 2010 annual report. It's a compelling theory: inject new stem cells into the brain, and they will grow new neurons. But when researchers at Stanford injected stem cells into the brains of rats that had been damaged by stroke, only half of these stem cells became new neurons and wired themselves into the networks of the rodents' brains—enough to make only a tiny functional difference.

But many of the rats showed dramatic recoveries, moving limbs that had previously been paralyzed by stroke. Certainly, the benefit of these stem cells went beyond their limited ability to patch the holes in the rats' neural networks.

Instead, or in addition, the stem cells seemed to respond to the damaged brains' calls for help with another kind of aid. In stroke or other brain damage, the brain's attempts at repair are frequently overwhelmed by the injury—the brain calls for help, but the few existing neural stem cells can't provide it in enough quantity to fix the damage. Plus, a stroke sets off a wave of secondary injuries, including inflammation, swelling, blood vessel spasms, and the accumulation of toxic cellular debris. But in these Stanford rats, the influx of new stem cells allowed them to turn the tide of injury, repairing the brain faster than it deteriorated. The CIRM article said, "The result: reduced inflammation, increased blood supply, new growth on existing neurons and new neuronal connections."

In other words, while the new stem cells didn't themselves function as the Army Corps of Engineers, they supplied the brain's existing engineers with the food, water, incentives, and perhaps raw materials they needed in order to work quickly and efficiently at their repair job.

Also, while injected stem cells didn't themselves generate new neurons, they promoted the growth of connections between the remaining neurons. Imagine pruning a road from a neighborhood map—replacing it with many small connections between side streets may allow cars to pass through the system just as quickly. And that's what stem cells did in these stroke-damaged rats—very few new neurons, but many connections that support the existing signals that flow through the brain.

And it seems as if, like Sigmund Freud's lying-on-the-couch treatment of psychiatric patients in the late 1800s, the benefit of stem cells injected into the brain may be a "talking cure." Do stem cells really talk the brain into repairing itself? Stanford professor of neurosurgery Gary Steinberg tested the theory by taping stem cells' mouths shut—figuratively speaking, of course.

The cancer drug Avastin blocks a messenger called vascular endothelial growth factor (VEGF), which commonly signals certain cells—such as blood vessel cells—to divide and grow. Blocking this communication in a cancer patient means that this growth factor can't promote the formation of blood vessels a tumor needs to grow. When Steinberg injected stroke-damaged rat brains with Avastin along with stem cells, the stem cells retained their limited ability to differentiate into neurons, but with their communication abilities muted—without the ability to spike this growth factor in the areas *around* damaged brain cells—many of the stem cells' positive effects disappeared.

Rather than the simple mechanism of stem cells equaling new brain tissue, the benefit of stem cells in the damaged brain seems mostly because of their ability to seek damage and generate a complex cocktail of biological agents that promote repair. Rather than the cavalry, they're more like battlefield medics, offering what scientists call paracrine effects (see chapter 2).

According to the CIRM 2010 annual report, Steinberg's group recently opened enrollment in a phase I "safety" trial using MSCs—bone-marrow-derived mesenchymal stem cells—which surgeons will implant in patients who experienced a stroke between six months and a year ago. The CIRM news release states, "In a previous small trial using these cells, there were no adverse effects, and some participants saw improvements in movement, memory, and spatial processing."

Of the clinical trial, Steinberg said, "I believe that stem cell transplantation for stroke holds great promise. Over the next probably two decades we will see remarkable advances."

The biotechnology company Aldagen is also exploring stem cells for use with stroke victims. In the fall of 2011 it started enrolling patients into a phase II clinical trial of its stem cell product ALD-401 (clinicaltrials.gov locator number NCT01273337). Injected into mice two weeks after a stroke, ALD-401 led to a 41 percent improvement in motor function compared to only an 11 percent improvement in untreated mice.

K. Jason Holly eagerly awaits these treatments. Jason earned a BA and an MBA from Stanford University and spent a successful thirty-year career as CEO of multiple technology companies. "I had my stroke on Thanksgiving morning, 2003," he says. The stroke paralyzed his right side, leaving him unable to swallow or speak. He was fifty-six years old. In a CIRM video, Jason, a fit-looking man now in his early sixties, overenunciates each word, punctuating his speech with chops from his left hand that land each phrase as if hammering nails. You can tell that it takes every fiber of his concentration to form the words, but you can also tell that behind the somewhat unwieldy musculature is a fully functioning intellect and a wonderful sense of humor.

As part of his recovery, Jason's wife, Mika, "tried singing 'Happy Birthday' with me—but we gave up on that because she has a terrible voice," he says, getting laughs from the crowd. "My wife did not give up on me, and I shared in her determination." He describes taking walks with his wife those days in the hospital: "I would give her my cane, after we passed the nurse's station, and just walk along holding on to her hand for balance." He was released from the hospital on Christmas Eve, 2003, and calls it "the best Christmas present I was ever given."

About six months after his stroke, Jason, a resident of the San Francisco Bay Area, walked the 7.5-mile Bay to Breakers Race, saying that he had run it for twenty years before his stroke and didn't want to lose his unbroken record. "My wife, who usually ran with me, didn't do this one," says Jason. "She said if I wanted to kill myself, I could do it without her present."

Even without stem cell treatment, Jason is a stroke success story—a testament to the power of a wife's faith and traditional rehabilitation medicine performed with tenacity and perseverance. But imagining a day in which, after a stroke, he not only walks but runs the Bay to Breakers Race, in which he returns to his career as a tech CEO, and in which he jokes effortlessly in front of a room of doctors isn't difficult.

The experimental treatment that very likely protected Jackson Dwyer's poststroke brain and that repaired the stroke-damaged brains of mice in Gary Steinberg's lab at Stanford is quickly moving its way into the clinic. In fact, in the United Kingdom, the treatment has already cleared the first hurdle—that of a phase I clinical trial, like the one Steinberg is just starting at Stanford. The University of Glasgow completed a safety trial of the procedure and is moving to the next step—trying to prove the treatment's effectiveness.

As we saw in the chapter on heart disease, in which three seemingly similar stem cell treatments for three seemingly similar conditions in fact turn out to be very different procedures aimed at very different ailments, not all stroke patients are created equal—and so different stem cell therapies may be appropriate for use with different patients. For example, in Jackson Dwyer's case, mesenchymal stem cells from the bone marrow of his hip likely helped *protect* his assaulted neurons from dying—the growth factors and other bio-protective ingredients they released near damaged (but not yet dead!) tissues likely stopped the progress of the damage and roused his brain to heal itself.

In contrast, the Glasgow study, named PISCES (for Pilot Investigation of Stem Cells in Stroke), is aimed at stroke victims of K. Jason Holly's type—patients whose ischemic stroke leaves completely dead brain tissue in its wake. Rather than protecting the brain with MSCs, PISCES hopes to regenerate dead tissue by injecting neural stem cells. And rather than harvesting and purifying a patient's own mesenchymal stem cells, the Glasgow trial is testing the injection of neural stem cells taken from a cell line they've grown in the lab. It's like making bread from a sourdough starter—when a patient needs the product, the university simply skims off a dose of neural stem cells from its lab-grown culture.

Treatment with a patient's own cells is called autologous and is in many ways easier than allogeneic treatment, or treatment with cells from a donor or from the lab. Autologous cells are unlikely to be rejected by a patient's body. But allogeneic, lab-grown cells offer the opportunity to have an off-the-shelf product that can potentially be administered soon after an ischemic head injury or stroke to prevent against any continuing damage—kind of like a cellular Advil. Then, goes the theory, a patient's own, autologous stem cells could be harvested, concentrated, and later infused in a way that provides the long-term engraftment needed to promote continued regeneration of damaged tissues.

In any case, a press release for the Glasgow study calls the neural stem cell product being tested a "clinical and commercial-grade cell therapy product capable of treating all eligible patients presenting." And it works in the lab. The university writes that the therapy "has been shown to reverse the functional deficits associated with stroke disability when administered several weeks after the stroke event in relevant models of the condition." This is science-ese for "It did great in mice."

The difference between "reverse" in this study and "protect" in earlier studies is a big one. It means that for patients like Jackson Dwyer, who was likely rescued from neural death by his own stem cells, the treatment was aimed at limiting ongoing brain damage and stimulating repair and regeneration in the time right after his injury. For patients like K. Jason Holly, the goal is to repair damage that has already happened and is now stable. Could his brain soon be brought back to life? In 2014, we should know definitively whether an injection of lab-grown neural stem cells can regenerate a dead brain.

But stroke is not the only way brain tissue dies. In many ways, cerebral palsy is its childhood equivalent. Unlike its name seems to imply, cerebral palsy is more a condition than a disease, resulting from mechanical difficulties in the womb or in the period surrounding birth that momentarily or chronically cut the brain's oxygen supply or otherwise injure the developing brain, leading to tissue death. Unlike stroke, which can usually be localized to a pinpoint area of the brain and so might neatly snip very specific functions like speech or movement on one side of the body, cerebral palsy tends to (but doesn't always) result in a broader brain injury. Common causes include brain infections while in the womb, an umbilical cord wrapped around a baby's neck at birth, or choking on toys while very young.

Neither parents nor doctors knew the cause of Houston

Crawford's cerebral palsy. But at two years old, after missing milestones like walking and talking, there it was: Houston was diagnosed with cerebral palsy. But his mother, Cynthia, remembered that they had banked baby Houston's umbilical cord blood when he was born—a smart move, as it turned out. Having this blood allowed them to take part in a Duke University clinical trial exploring the effect of autologous (remember: from a patient's own body) stem cells in children with cerebral palsy. Houston's blood stem cells were concentrated from the umbilical cord blood his parents had banked and were then infused through an IV into his blood in a procedure that lasted less than an hour.

Five days later, Houston spoke his first words. His dad grabbed a video camera, and the footage became part of a 2008 *Today* show report that's easy to find with a quick online search. After his treatment, Houston also started waving and laughing, and, according to his parents, he appeared more curious. "It seemed like a fog was over him before," Houston's mom told Meredith Vieira on *Today*, "and now you can't get anything past him. He's just very smart. Before he went to Duke, we were trying to teach him to use a walker, and now he walks with no assistance at all. To us it's just amazing."

Yes, this is anecdotal evidence. And yes, a creative mind can come up with other explanations for Houston's improvement. And yes, more scientific investigation is required to understand exactly what happened and whether Houston's results are likely in other patients. But the anecdotal evidence is pretty compelling. In the *Today* video, the homemade clip of Houston shows him grabbing a table for support as he looks toward the camera and says, "Mamma, Mamma!"

Cynthia started a website to raise money for families exploring similar treatments. She wrote in November 2010 that

"Houston is starting swim lessons and soccer league this summer, and he is very excited! So proud of him!!!"

A miracle happened to Houston Crawford. Following the Duke study, the Medical College of Georgia has recently started its own clinical trial to delve into the cause of this miracle. Like Duke, the trial explores the effects of (banked) autologous umbilical-cord-blood stem cells with cerebral palsy patients. But unlike the Duke study, instead of simply giving stem cells to check that the procedure is safe (the first phase of any FDA-approved clinical trial), this follow-up is a "double blind placebo controlled trial"—one group of children gets stem cells, and one group initially gets a placebo. Even doctors don't know which patients are in the experimental group. With a neurological exam up front and then another neurological exam three months after treatment, researchers should be able to discover which of the 40 children improved and which did not. (At that point, children who got a placebo will also be infused with their cord-blood stem cells, so both the experimental and control groups eventually get the real treatment.)

If you have or know of a child with banked umbilical cord blood who might benefit from this stem cell treatment of cerebral palsy, consider searching for trial number NCT01072370 at http://www.clinicaltrials.gov. Families in the study can also apply for full or partial grants to cover travel expenses through the Newborn Possibilities Fund, a philanthropic arm of the Cord Blood Registry. Any results are still firmly in the realm of *maybe*—the treatment may or may not work—but so far it looks like it has a chance.

If stroke is primarily a disease of the aged and cerebral palsy is primarily a disease of the young, then traumatic brain injury (TBI) is the umbrella that covers them both. TBI can happen at any age.

Perhaps the most famous case of traumatic brain injury is that of Phineas Gage. As a twenty-five-year-old in 1848, Gage was using a tamping rod to pack gunpowder into a hole as part of a railroad construction project when the gunpowder exploded, blasting the three-foot-long pointed metal rod backward toward him. The missile smashed through his head underneath his left eye, passed through his brain, and exited the top of his skull, behind and above his right eye.

Amazingly, Gage survived the accident. The physician John Harlow stabilized Gage after the accident and then monitored not only his physical recovery but also the changes to the psychological and emotional person that was Phineas Gage. Gage kept his abilities to walk and talk, and his IQ was unchanged. But according to an article on the National Institutes of Health website, "Before the accident Gage was a quiet, mild-mannered man; after his injuries he became an obscene, obstinate, self-absorbed man. He continued to suffer personality and behavioral problems until his death in 1861." The tamping rod had chopped the part of Gage's brain responsible for "executive function," leaving him without a check-and-balance for his impulses.

In the United States, TBI affects mostly male teenagers and young adults aged fifteen to twenty-four and children younger than five. As you might have guessed, these are the people most likely to hit their heads on things. Half of all TBIs are caused by motor vehicle accidents, commonly involving motorcycles, and half of all TBIs are alcohol-related. Of course, like cerebral palsy and stroke, there is a huge spectrum of TBI ranging from a mild concussion with no lasting effects to a fatal gunshot wound. TBI may also increase the later risk and onset of neurodegenerative diseases like Alzheimer's and Parkinson's (as seen in the boxer Muhammad Ali).

Michael Alman's brain injury was the result of jumping off a boat. A native of Delray Beach, Florida, in 2002 Michael dove off the back of his boat into unexpectedly shallow water and hit his head on the bottom. When he wasn't pulled out in time, he nearly drowned, which, even in correct medical terminology, "added insult to injury."

Michael's traumatic brain injury was extensive. After being placed in a medically induced coma, he woke up months later, connected to a ventilator and unable to see. He was paralyzed from the chest down.

Michael decided to fly to China for experimental stem cell treatment. These overseas treatments aren't covered by insurance, so Michael's church worked hard to raise the nearly $40,000 he needed for treatment. In a blog about his experiences (http://stemcellschina.com/blog/david/), Michael writes that before he left, his church "dedicated part of the service and a hymn to my farewell while Mom and Dad were there. It was moving and brought tears to all of us. I am incredibly blessed to have a church family as wonderful as them. I am so grateful to everyone for their generosity and messages of hope and prayer."

A documentary team from National Geographic Channel followed Michael to China, where he was treated with stem cells harvested from a placenta after the birth of a Chinese baby. "Right now this is where hope is. This is where you come for hope. This is where our future is. Right now this is the only thing we have that we can hold on to," Michael told the camera team, his speech slurring through the viscous oil that is his injury. Despite the expense and American researchers' misgivings, Michael and other patients in the National Geographic documentary *Supercell* express their opinions that for their conditions, some hope of improvement is worth the cost and risk.

Did Michael stand from his wheelchair and walk unassisted onto the airplane back to the United States? No. But he told

Florida's WPBF that "while I was there, the third week, things started to come more into view. I started being able to read things." Before his treatment, he was blind. Afterward, he said, he could see. Michael also credited the stem cell therapy with improving his motor control. In *Supercell*, an extremely pleased Michael rocks forward in his wheelchair and then leans back. He does it again and again and explains to the camera that this movement is a new development—and that it's only the start. Michael hopes that strengthening the muscles in his trunk will one day allow him to walk.

In its own way, this video of Michael Alman is equal parts inspirational and cautionary. It depicts someone looking with hope into a brighter tomorrow—a tomorrow that's still a long ways off and which, perhaps, for Michael, may never come. Or it might. Michael writes that after being completely blind in 2002, in 2009 after two trips to China, his vision improved to 20/50 in his left eye and 20/30 in his right. The blog also shows his attempts to stand from a seated position, with the help of "a new therapist who is 6'5" and strong enough to handle my weight," he said. On the tape, Michael says he can't do it. He pushes. His legs and arms shake. With help, he stands. Then, when his therapist asks him to sit, Michael hesitates—it's as if he doesn't want to lower back to his seat, as if he knows he can stand another couple seconds, as if for a few short seconds he remembers what his legs used to be.

Almost all the scientists quoted in this book believe Michael's improvement and the gains of almost all patients at these overseas stem cell clinics are because of the awesome power of renewed hope and not the stem cell treatments themselves. This book includes very few case studies involving these clinics, but this one is included in hopes that it will help you make up your own mind.

Current FDA-approved stem cell treatments for brain conditions, including stroke, cerebral palsy, and traumatic brain injury, are showing *initial* promise. In these clinical trials, there are legitimate success stories. There is hope. But there's a long road ahead between the landmark stories of Houston Crawford's cerebral palsy and Jackson Dwyer's stroke and what most people would call a cure.

Right now, these treatments are tipping from theory to practice. And even if stem cells aren't themselves the agents of improvement in some of these overseas clinics, after treatment Michael Alman gained the ability to drive his powered wheelchair around his neighborhood. "Being able to take my dog out for a walk every day is the best part of my life," he said, and though science is skeptical, Michael attributes this best part of his life to stem cell therapy.

Chapter 5

Psychiatric Disorders

Heinz Prechter's earliest memories were of crouching behind the heavy wooden door of his family's German farmhouse as Allied planes flew overhead in the closing months of World War II. In 1963, at age twenty-one, Heinz came to the United States to study business at San Francisco State College. He earned tuition by installing sunroofs, which were then a brand-new, custom invention. Fifteen months later, Heinz dropped out of school. He spent $764 on tools, made a workbench from an old door, scavenged a sewing machine from a junkyard, and founded the American Sunroof Company.

The company Heinz founded now has more than one thousand employees across the United States. Among many other awards, he earned the prestigious Entrepreneur of the Year award from the Harvard Business Club.

On July 6, 2001, Heinz Prechter hung himself in the pool house of his home in Grosse Ile, Michigan.

Throughout his adult life, Heinz had suffered with bouts of manic depression. Finally, it killed him. "He had this gift, and at the same time he had this burden," his widow, Wally Prechter, told the *Detroit News*. In Matthew 17:15, some people believe

the Apostle Matthew refers to manic depression, or as psychia-
trists now call it, bipolar disorder, when he writes: "Lord, have
mercy on my son: for he is a lunatic and he falleth into the
fire, and oft into the water." With the help of Wally Prechter's
foundation, established at the University of Michigan after her
husband's death, stem cells may someday help patients afflicted
with manic depression walk a middle path between fire and water, avoiding this cruel psychiatric affliction.

And so unlike previous chapters, this is one about what stem
cells could be. They aren't there yet, but if you or a loved one
suffers from bipolar disorder, schizophrenia, depression, or one
of many other psychiatric disorders, know that there's hope.
And this cutting-edge hope is coming from the stem cells of
psychiatric patients themselves.

Researchers have linked cancer, Huntington's disease, multiple sclerosis, cystic fibrosis, spina bifida, and more than one
thousand other conditions to the genes that either cause them or
predispose one to them. Finding these genes allows researchers
to do two very important things: explore how turning these
genes on or off affects the disease as well as study these genes in
cells or mice (sometimes artificially inserted) in order to study
the disease process and test drugs.

So far, even after extensive searching, no one has been able to
nail down the genes that cause bipolar disorder.

Generally, to discover the cause of a genetic disease, researchers compare healthy cells to diseased cells and see what's
different. Of course, to do this, you need samples of healthy and
affected tissue. And unfortunately, it's not easy to sample people's brains. Even outside the question of what removing a small
chunk of brain tissue might do to the patient, the mechanics of
sampling the brain are tricky. Mostly, that's because the brain
is protected by the thick barrier of the dura, which helps keep

infection out—and doctors don't poke through the dura without very good reason. Certainly, the desire for a sample of a schizo- phrenic or bipolar person's brain tissue isn't a good enough reason. Not to mention that it's unclear what area or areas of the brain are abnormal in various mental illnesses, making it unclear where you would even take a sample from.

And so it's hard to get enough samples from enough people with psychiatric disorders to draw any meaningful conclusions about what in their brains creates their conditions.

"Currently, the best treatments for bipolar disorder are only effective for 30 percent to 50 percent of patients," says Dr. Melvin McInnis, associate director of the University of Michi- gan Depression Center. "New discoveries have been limited, in part due to the lack of access to tissue and cells from individuals with bipolar disorder. But that is now changing because of the Prechter research program and advances in stem cell research."

Basically, University of Michigan scientists discovered how to create bipolar brain cells from the skin stem cells of psychi- atric patients. It starts with a tiny skin sample, which you'll note is a lot easier to get than brain tissue. Scientists pull out the skin stem cells and then inject them with genes that wipe away their developmental past, returning these cells to an embryonic- like state. These induced pluripotent stem cells sometimes form tumors when used for treatments, but they're spectacular for generating cells that scientists can experiment on.

"We often think of stem cells being used in therapies to treat disease, but this is a great example of stem cells' usefulness for studying the mechanisms of disease," says Sue O'Shea, PhD, di- rector of the University of Michigan Consortium for Stem Cell Therapies. Because these induced pluripotent cells renew them- selves, a small sample of these engineered cells can give rise to a line of cells that researchers can keep incubating in the lab and skim as needed for experimentation. A tiny patch of a bipolar patient's skin can create the brain cells that hold the genetic secrets of their disease, or rule out a genetic basis and help researchers focus their efforts on finding environmental or other acquired causes.

The University of Michigan team is using induced pluripotent stem cells to create thirty of these cell lines, ten from healthy volunteers and twenty from patients with bipolar disorder. What's different between these bipolar and healthy cell lines? Now, finally, researchers will have the samples they need to discover the genetic underpinnings of this disease.

In April 2011, researchers at the Salk Institute for Biological Studies did almost exactly the same thing with schizophrenia. "Nobody knows how much the environment contributes to the disease," study researcher Kristen Brennand, a postdoctoral researcher at Salk, told the science news site LiveScience. "By growing neurons in a dish, we can take the environment out of the equation and start focusing on the underlying biological problems."

One thing growing these petri dish populations of schizophrenic brain cells shows is that there are fewer connections between these cells than in dishes of healthy cells grown in the same way. Salk researchers also found six hundred genes that seemed to be doing different things in the schizophrenic cells. More samples grown from the skin of more schizophrenic patients are needed to narrow down this list to the prime offenders.

The magazine *Scientific American* reported in 2006 that stem cell treatment for depression is further along.

To understand depression, we must start with the hippocampus—the little seahorse-shaped region in your brain responsible for taking in new memories. The hippocampus is one of only two brain structures whose stem cells continue to make new neurons throughout adulthood. Research in the mid-2000s showed that the hippocampi of depressed mice and monkeys make fewer new neurons than their happier peers. Antidepressants reverse this trend, increasing the growth of new neurons in the hippocampus by 75 percent or more.

So, by the late 2000s, researchers were pretty convinced that lack of stem cell activity in the hippocampus creates depression—no new neurons made sad animals, and new neurons made happy ones . . . at least as happy and sad as we can tell in mice and monkeys.

Scientific American described the coffin nail: scientists from Columbia University and Yale zapped the hippocampi of depressed mice with radiation so that they couldn't make new neurons. Then, when these mice got antidepressants, the drugs didn't work. If an antidepressant couldn't stimulate stem cells in the hippocampus to make new neurons, the rodents stayed depressed.

The *Scientific American* article added, "If neurogenesis is required to kick depression, as the result suggested, maybe its loss sends the mind into a tailspin."

It also implies a possible cure: if lack of stem cell activity in the hippocampus causes depression, perhaps injecting new neural stem cells into this system would cure it. Could this technique have saved Heinz Prechter or the more than 90 percent of suicides that are associated with depression and related disorders (according to the National Institute of Mental Health)?

Researchers don't know yet.

But already this speculative work with stem cells has made one hugely important difference in patients' lives.

Fred Gage, a professor at the Salk Institute's Laboratory of Genetics, told LiveScience that before this research, "many people believed that if affected individuals just worked through their problems, they could overcome them. But we are showing real biological dysfunctions in neurons that are independent of the environment."

While stem cells don't yet offer a cure for psychiatric illnesses, they show that the disorders are every bit as real as cancer or other chronic illnesses, so, like drugs, stem cell interventions have to combat the biology of these diseases of the brain. Plus, who's to say that "talk therapy," perhaps by stimulating underused brain connections, doesn't somehow spur those dormant, depressed stem cells into action, getting them to start making new neurons?

Stem cells can't yet cure depression, but they can cure how society treats depressed people.

Chapter 6

Spinal Cord Injuries

Eli is a donkey. And like most donkeys, online video footage of Eli shows that rather than being "good," Eli is what you'd call "full of personality." He's obstinate and cock-eared and undeniably lovable in the manner of a mad child who acts cute without wanting to.

Like the donkey that Jesus rode humbly into Jerusalem for his entrance into Jerusalem (Matthew 21:1–11), Eli is a small donkey, a burro, and until 2010 he lived with his friend, Watson, a "jack" donkey almost twice Eli's size. Until the morning of May 13, 2010, they seemed best friends. But on that morning, inexplicably, Watson bit Eli on the neck and shook him like a dog with a chew toy. The attack snapped Eli's neck back and forth. While Eli didn't go down as if his legs had been cut from underneath him, continued swelling in his spinal cord saw the little donkey deteriorate over the next couple days. His legs got weaker. On May 18, five days after the attack, Eli went to a special equine hospital for treatment.

"We did a normal treatment of anti-inflammatories and hyperbaric oxygen therapy, but he was deteriorating very fast right in front of us," veterinarian Doug Herthel, the equine hospital's founder and chief of staff, told a reporter from *Horse and Man* magazine.

On May 22, an MRI showed that the attack had resulted in swelling that was squeezing the life out of little Eli's spinal cord. His prognosis was poor. By May 24, he was paralyzed in all four limbs, couldn't lift his head, and couldn't urinate or defecate. Eli had also developed pneumonia.

On May 25, Herthel presented Eli's owner with two options: euthanasia or an experimental stem cell treatment. In fact, Herthel was a pioneer in stem cell treatments for horses, having used them to treat nearly five thousand horses for tendon and ligament damage. But this was different—he'd never before used stem cells for spinal injury. In fact, to his knowledge, no one had.

The theory made sense. Stem cells are known to do two relevant things: promote angiogenesis (the formation of new blood vessels) and decrease inflammation—both of which likely helped protect Jackson Dwyer's brain after stroke, as seen in chapter 4.

With nothing to lose, Eli's owner and Herthel decided to give it a try.

That morning of May 25, as Eli lay paralyzed and dying of pneumonia, Herthel injected the little donkey's spinal column with 70 million mesenchymal stem cells banked from a thoroughbred horse.

Within forty-eight hours, Eli started moving.

"Eli's owner drove sixty miles round-trip daily to visit him and to provide lots of carrots, horse cookies, and TLC," Herthel told *Horse and Man*. By June 8, Eli could stand in his stall with help. Then, after a second injection of stem cells, again within forty-eight hours, Eli showed a leap in improvement, taking a couple steps on his own. On June 20, Eli got a third and final injection of mesenchymal stem cells from the thoroughbred donor, and on July 2, he was able to roll up onto his chest.

Eli the donkey continued to improve, and on July 31, Herthel found Eli standing in his stall. "We couldn't figure out how he got up," Herthel told *Horse and Man*. "So we went back and looked at the video, and we saw him get up on his own. It wasn't pretty, but he got up, and that's what counts. After that third treatment, he just got better and better, and his muscle mass came back." A quick online search shows video of Eli the donkey standing for the first time.

Eventually Eli was released from Herthel's equine hospital and returned to his Santa Barbara–area ranch, where his improvement continued. The article in *Horse and Man* doesn't mention whether Eli was reunited with Watson, but we imagine not.

Some professional observers of this account of healing point to the fact that Eli's spinal cord was only compressed and not actually severed. These doctors and researchers say that Eli's recovery was due to decreased swelling around the spinal column and not to the growth and reconnection of spinal cord fibers across a break. And they're right. But even after aggressive treatment with traditional medicine, Eli was deteriorating, and anti-inflammatories had failed to allow the spinal cord to heal.

Stem cells did.

No, this story does not prove that stem cells are effective in healing spinal cord tears. But the point is this: in Eli's case, stem cells were a new, better anti-inflammatory drug, and they provided aid to spinal cord tissue that would otherwise have been missing. No, stem cells didn't "repair" a tear in Eli's spinal cord, but the fact remains that the stem cell therapy likely saved his life—again, cellular Advil to the rescue.

That said, new science shows that the big prize—repair after spinal cord tear—may be within reach. In December 2010, Japanese researchers injected induced pluripotent stem cells—adult skin cells that had been genetically reprogrammed to return them to an embryonic-like state—into a marmoset that was paralyzed from the neck down.

"It is the world's first case in which a small-size primate recovered from a spinal injury using stem cells," Professor Hideyuki Okano of Tokyo's Keio University told the *American Free Press*.

In this study, Okano and colleagues injected the induced pluripotent cells into the marmoset nine days after injury, and then, after six weeks, the marmoset was "jumping around," Okano says. The doctor says that the marmoset regained up to 80 percent of the gripping strength in its forefeet.

As with many therapies described in this book, the United States is just now starting to push past these animal models into clinical trials of stem cells to treat spinal cord injuries, while in other countries, versions of the therapy are already in human use. A quick Google search finds clinics in China, India, and Portugal willing—for a price—to inject stem cells into the damaged tissues of spinal cord injury patients.

And some of these clinics have even published their safety results in respected medical journals. For example, take the results from a study in India's Nichi-In Centre for Regenerative Medicine, published in 2008 in the peer-reviewed journal *Cell Transplantation*, which states, "To date, we have administered BMSCs [bone marrow stem cells] into 52 patients with SCI [spinal cord injury] and have had no tumor formations, no cases of infection or increased pain, and few instances of minor adverse events. These studies demonstrate that BMSCs administration via multiple routes is feasible, safe, and may improve the quality of life for patients living with spinal cord injury."

There are two important takeaways from this careful language: the first is the clinic's impeccable safety record, and the second is the word *may* in the final sentence. In almost all publications in peer-reviewed journals, the evidence is that stem cell treatments in India, China, Portugal, and elsewhere for spinal cord injuries are safe and "may" improve quality of life. The evidence of benefit is anecdotal, meaning that patients may report improvements, but these gains either haven't been verified by tests or can't be necessarily linked to stem cell treatments. By the end of this book, this warning might sound like a broken record, but the fact remains: there is very little evidence that these overseas stem cell clinics provide any real benefit for spinal cord injuries outside the gains generated by renewed hope and aggressive rehabilitation therapy.

Still, the stories are compelling. Here is a story that puts a foot on either side of the fence that divides controlled clinical trials in research hospitals from anecdotal evidence of miracle cures in private clinics.

The first United States citizen to receive a stem cell treatment in Portugal for spinal cord injury was Siri Moor. In October 2001, Siri and her brother went for a fast-food run after a party for their parents' twenty-fifth wedding anniversary in Farmington Hills, Michigan. On that night, in their suburb, twenty-three-year-old Siri's car flipped off the road and the airbag went off. Somehow she bent her neck against this airbag, snapping her spine and the cord within it at the C6 vertebrae, low in her cervical spine. On the scale of spinal injuries, Siri's fracture was designated a dire "Asia A." She was paralyzed from her chest down, able only to move her right arm slightly.

"By the grace of God, I pray that your family will never know this experience," her dad said in testimony before the Michigan House of Representatives.

Two years later, traditional rehabilitation therapy had produced negligible results. "I was in a power wheelchair," Siri told the magazine *New Mobility*. "It took me a month to learn to feed myself."

It was then that Siri and her parents began exploring other options. And now is when many cooks join the kitchen of this story. Associate Professor Jean Peduzzi-Nelson, of the Department of Anatomy and Cell Biology at Wayne State University in Detroit, is no stranger to stem cells—she's testified three times in front of the United States Congress about the benefits and potential benefits of adult, autologous (from the patient) stem cell therapies. It's only twenty-four miles along Highway 10 from Siri's family home in Farmington Hills to the Wayne State University School of Medicine, and so the pairing of injured Siri Moor with Dr. Peduzzi-Nelson was a natural one.

Unfortunately, after unsuccessful rehabilitation therapy under Peduzzi-Nelson's care, Siri continued to lack the dramatic results she wanted. But Peduzzi-Nelson had been working to design a stem cell spinal cord study with Dr. Carlos Lima, a researcher in Lisbon, Portugal, where the clinical use of stem cells is a little less tightly regulated. If Siri received treatment in Lisbon, after returning home she would add another member to her team, Dr. Steven Hinderer, specialist-in-chief at the Rehabilitation Institute of Michigan in Detroit, who would oversee her continuing rehabilitation.

Peduzzi-Nelson was a leading stem cell lab researcher, Lima was a leading spinal surgeon, and Hinderer was a top-notch rehabilitation specialist. If anything could work, Siri Moor thought, this would be it.

In 2003, Siri traveled to Lisbon's Egas Moniz Hospital for

the five-hour procedure. First, Dr. Lima and his surgical team opened her spinal column to clear away scar tissue and skeletal debris. Then they went after her stem cells.

As you know by now, stem cells are found in many places in the human body. Really, most tissues that die or are killed over time have a corresponding stem cell population that replenishes them. For example, because blood cells are constantly dying, stem cells in human bone marrow are constantly making new blood. As you also know by now, these bone marrow stem cells are primarily what we call mesenchymal stem cells, and these MSCs can create a number of tissues, including blood, bones, cartilage, and fat. But (again, as we've seen), while they can and do make nerve cells, MSCs aren't optimized for it. Rather than transforming into new neurons in the brains of stroke and traumatic brain injury victims, the healing power of these MSCs seems due more to the growth factors and other bio-protective and bio-regenerative signals they produce when they encounter distressed cells.

To heal a severed spinal cord, Peduzzi-Nelson, Lima, Hinderer, and especially Siri Moor would need something more than stem cell signaling and support. They would need tissue growth. And so instead of using mesenchymal stem cells from the bone marrow of Siri's hip, as had been done in previous nervous system studies, Peduzzi-Nelson and the Portuguese doctors used cells that had already taken a small step forward from their MSC parents toward nervous tissue.

The primary olfactory receptor neurons in your nose don't have the body's cushiest job. In fact, a 2007 article in the journal *Nature Neuroscience* describes how, as you breathe, these unfortunate nasal nerve fibers are constantly bombarded by "pathogens and other noxious substances," which leads to bad things like dying. And so, just as your body replenishes blood, it has a built-in method of replenishing dead primary olfactory receptor neurons. In fact, there's a population of stem cells that the body puts in charge of regenerating these neurons.

If this sounds promising, that's because it is. Unlike MSCs, these olfactory receptor neuron stem cells are already optimized to create nervous tissue. And so after cleaning the debris from Siri's spinal column, Dr. Lima and his team inserted a thin tube into her nose to harvest a population of these stem cells. Surgeons then cut the olfactory tissue into small pieces and soaked it in Siri's cerebrospinal fluid—the nutrient bathwater of the brain and spinal cord. Then they opened up one of the empty pockets in her spine—a cyst where tissue death had left a fluid-filled space—and injected this material, rich with nervous system stem cells, into the void. Would the treatment fill this void with functioning tissue? Time would tell.

Siri went back to Detroit, back to Hinderer, who, contrary to what his name may imply, was meant to whip her recovery into gear. For five hours a day, three days a week (and two hours a day on her "off days"), Siri worked to move and to stretch, gaining muscle and confidence. She learned to move her fingers and can now lift a water bottle to drink. She learned to move her arms and can now push herself up off an exercise ball. The magazine *New Mobility* reported that her sensory restoration is evident down to about what is called the T10 level, a full 11 spinal levels below the site of her C6 injury.

Her recovery has been so extensive that Siri left her motorized wheelchair behind. In *New Mobility* she wrote, "Now I use a TiLite titanium rigid frame chair. If there's something that's really steep up or down I still need assistance, but for the most part I can maneuver just fine." With leg braces, a walker, and a therapist, she can even approximate walking on a treadmill.

In 2006, three years after her surgery, Siri went back to Portugal for a follow-up with Dr. Lima. During that visit, Dr. Lima used magnetic resonance imaging (MRI) to peer into the pocket that was Siri's cyst. Where before there was a void, now there were new blood vessels and, presumably, synapses.

Since starting with Portuguese patients in 2001 and then with Siri in 2003, Dr. Lima has performed 120-and-counting similar operations, a number that's starting to generate some compelling data. This is where Peduzzi-Nelson, the researcher from Wayne State University, comes back into this story. In January 2010, based on twenty patients who were treated as a group along with Siri, Lima and Peduzzi-Nelson published the study's findings in the respected journal *Neurorehabilitation and Neural Repair*, which you can find by searching for the study's title, "Olfactory Mucosal Autografts and Rehabilitation for Chronic Traumatic Spinal Cord Injury."

How did these twenty subjects fare?

Before treatment, all twenty had total paralysis below the level of their spinal cord injuries. The Wayne State University news release said, "One paraplegic treated almost three years after the injury now ambulates [walks] with two crutches and knee braces. Ten other patients ambulate with physical assistance and walkers (with and without braces). One 31-year-old male [quadriplegic] patient uses a walker without the help of knee braces or physical assistance." Overall, a majority of the patients in the study showed significant improvement in their responses and clinical test scores.

"This may be the first clinical study of patients with severe, chronic spinal cord injury to report considerable functional improvement in some patients with a combination treatment," Peduzzi-Nelson said. "Normally, in people with spinal cord injuries that happened more than eighteen months ago, there is little improvement."

Still, some chalk these improvements up to hope, belief, and the extremely aggressive rehabilitation therapy that accompanied the stem cell treatment. According to this line of reasoning, the benefit of this stem cell implantation is flipping the psychological switch into a mentality that believes that recovery is possible. These patients, the story goes, are more likely to aggressively pursue physical rehabilitation therapy, which is what creates these partial recoveries.

Drs. Peduzzi-Nelson and Lima are the first to admit that more study is needed. Even Siri's story of recovery and the many stories like hers are anecdotal and prone to multiple interpretations of what, exactly, caused the benefit—was it stem cells, or was it intensive rehabilitation?

Peduzzi-Nelson is happy to take on the challenge of teasing apart these two threads. Toward the goal of creating carefully designed clinical trials to remove the subjectivity from the study of stem cell treatments, in 2010 Peduzzi-Nelson helped found a program called ASCENT, which stands for Adult Stem Cells Engineered for Neural Therapy. The program hopes to soon bring olfactory mucosa stem cell therapies to clinical trial for stroke, brain injury, and chemotherapy-induced brain damage.

Other researchers are pursuing similar lines of study. As of the fall of 2011, ClinicalTrials.gov lists open clinical trials of mesenchymal stem cells with spinal cord injuries in Switzerland, China, Brazil, and the Institute for Rehabilitation and Research at the University of Texas Health Sciences Center (number NCT01328860).

As for Siri Moor, she takes her recovery one step at a time. Literally. After trading her motorized wheelchair for a human-powered one, Knight-Ridder newspapers report that she has now set her sights on walking. With a physical therapist supporting her from behind and calipers on her legs, Siri walks on a treadmill. Her weight has to be centered just right. Her back must be straight, with her feet just the right distance apart. She has to land on her heels, not her toes. And in this way she "walks."

Is it walking, or is it wishful thinking?

"It seems, just when I get discouraged, I feel or experience something new," Siri says. With or without walking, Siri's doctors call her recovery miraculous. With a host of studies springing from her early reports of success, perhaps we'll soon know if this miracle was due to stem cells.

Chapter 7

Alzheimer's, Parkinson's, and Other Neurodegenerative Diseases

Unlike the Grim Reaper's scythe of traumatic brain injury or stroke, neurodegenerative diseases can be a slow fade. And many of these diseases go beyond erasing memories—they can also erode emotion and personality until you or the one you love may bear little resemblance to the person you were or knew.

Having cared for his mother as she slipped into dementia, Joe Paula knew about Alzheimer's disease. "She wouldn't know who I was," Joe told the California Institute for Regenerative Medicine. "So when things started happening to me, I was very, very nervous. I really kind of kept it to myself." Joe started forgetting things. Eventually whole conversations slipped from his mind. Stretched out in front of him, Joe saw the road of decline, and it was a terrifying road he knew all too well.

Alzheimer's disease was first described in 1906 by the German psychologist and neuropathologist Alois Alzheimer. But despite its long history and more than 750 clinical trials aimed at the disease, scientists still aren't exactly sure what causes it.

Certainly one feature of Alzheimer's disease is the loss of connections between neurons, called synapses. Here's how it works: when a neuron "fires," it releases a chemical called

71

acetylcholine that jumps the small gap from the end of the first neuron to the beginning of the next. There are other "neurotransmitters," but for this example we'll stick with acetylcholine. The chain reaction continues, passing the signal from neuron to neuron through the brain. In healthy brains, this gap-jumping chemical is either quickly reabsorbed or destroyed by an enzyme called cholinesterase, among others. No worries; the brain can always create more signaling chemical, and it's best not to have stray chemicals bopping around the brain.

But the Alzheimer's brain can't make more. The disease reduces the brain's ability to produce the neurotransmitter acetylcholine and thus a neuron's ability to make the next neuron in the chain fire. Neurons that fire together, wire together—this is one of the basics of human learning—but the reverse is also true: neurons that don't successfully pass information through their synapses eventually lose these synapses. It's as if by not using these telephone lines, the lines are eventually pruned from the system. This keeps the healthy brain optimized but sends the Alzheimer's brain into decline. Lost synapses result in lost function.

There are drugs that target this synapse loss. Remember the natural enzyme that quickly destroys the neurotransmitter acetylcholine? There are drugs that keep this destruction from happening. In fact, these inhibitors were developed from snake venom and are commonly used as military nerve agents. In healthy brains, the inability to get rid of this neurotransmitter results in signal overload and quickly "fries" the brain. But administered at the right dose in the Alzheimer's brain, these inhibitors result in stronger signals and thus less synapse death.

As in all of medicine, there is a very fine line between medicine and poison.

And far from a magic bullet, according to the Alzheimer's

Association, these cholinesterase inhibitors delay the worsening of symptoms for six to twelve months in half of the patients who try them—a modest effect, at best.

Another theory about Alzheimer's disease is that a plaque forms around neurons, first slowing and eventually killing them—a bit like cholesterol choking blood vessels. This plaque is made of a protein fragment called amyloid beta. In a healthy brain, these protein fragments are broken down and eliminated. In Alzheimer's disease, the fragments accumulate to form hard, insoluble plaques.

Certainly more plaque is seen in the Alzheimer's brain. Science has shown that a certain gene predisposes some people to Alzheimer's disease and that people with this gene are also predisposed to plaque buildup in their brains. The question is, does this plaque *cause* Alzheimer's disease, or is it just the *result* of the *real* disease process in Alzheimer's? Unfortunately, it seems to be the latter—a 2004 study published in the journal *Neuron* showed little correlation between plaque buildup and neuron death. This is unfortunate, because in early human trials, a vaccine proved effective in reversing the course of this plaque buildup—but patients showed no improvement in their symptoms of dementia.

Perhaps a *third* theory of Alzheimer's will point the way toward a cure? In addition to the neurotransmitter theory and the plaque theory, scientists have added the tangle theory of the disease. Within neurons there are proteins called *tau* that form microtubules that function as tiny pipelines to transport nutrients and other vital substances throughout the nerve cell. The tangle theory holds that abnormal tau proteins start to fold back on themselves like sticky, overcooked pasta. This stickiness results in tubule tangles within the nerve fiber and eventually the death of these tissues.

Fourth and finally, some scientists think Alzheimer's may be caused by the breakdown of the fatty sheath that insulates neurons and thus allows them to contain their electric current. Breakdown of this myelin sheath lets electrical signals leak into the brain, and neurons that lose their ability to conduct electricity eventually die.

Again, these four things—tangles, plaque, lack of neurotransmitter, and myelin breakdown—are characteristics of Alzheimer's. But which, if any, is the cause? And which, when reversed or repaired, may be the cure?

No matter the cause and the cure, the reality is that right now the disease marches inexorably, like a million-strong school of army ants. So far, this school of ants has overwhelmed everything that science has put in front of it, spilling over the medical barricades and consuming everything in its path. As Alzheimer's grows, the brain shrinks. Short-term memory loss is followed by steeper cognitive decline and eventually by the shutdown of bodily functions and death.

Five percent of the United States' population shows symptoms of Alzheimer's disease at age sixty-five, and the number climbs to 25 percent at age eighty-five or older. The United Nations Department of Economic and Social Affairs estimates that in 2050, the disease will touch one in every eighty-five people on Earth. Adjusting for population, that will make more than 100 million worldwide sufferers, a staggering number that will swamp our health-care systems and our ability to care for our elders.

When he was diagnosed, Joe Paula said, "I really believed I was going to be going down like Mother, that I wouldn't know my children, and I wouldn't know my wife." He treated the disease with an off-label cholinesterase inhibitor and, in the short period after his diagnosis, has avoided steep cognitive decline.

But this barricade can last only so long—Joe is already past the one-year mark that's typically the top end of the drug's effectiveness. The dam's cement is cracking, and it's only a matter of time before leaks become a torrent.

But while science doesn't have an answer for Alzheimer's, medicine might—and there's an important difference to understand. Sometimes things just work. Sometimes, despite a lack of understanding of the underlying scientific mechanism, the medicine of stem cells just does its thing. Nature often achieves fixes that man cannot yet understand.

Frank LaFerla, PhD, director of the Institute for Memory Impairments and Neurological Disorders at the University of California, Irvine (UCI MIND), was a skeptic. He held little hope that stem cells could reverse the course of Alzheimer's, but he decided to let science, or nature, be the judge.

LaFerla had eighteen-month-old rats specially bred to develop plaque-ridden, myelin-deficient brains that appeared to mimic human Alzheimer's brains. He put the Alzheimer's rats in a water maze—a large tub with a hidden, small, circular platform where rats could haul themselves out. Over and over LaFerla put the Alzheimer's rats into the same maze, and again and again, they failed to learn where the platform was. The rats simply couldn't remember the path to safety, and each trip into the water maze was as if they were experiencing it for the first time. In contrast, normal rats quickly learned where safety lay.

The hippocampus is the area of both the rat and the human brains responsible for coding new memories. Information or experience hits the hippocampus, and the little brain region acts like a business's receiving dock—it accepts shipments and packages them for storage deeper in the brain. You might remember that the hippocampus is also one of the two areas in the adult brain that continues to make use of its stem cells throughout your life. The hippocampus is always growing new neurons. But in the Alzheimer's brain, the pace of growth doesn't match the pace of neural death.

So LaFerla gave these rats a boost, injecting their hippocampi with neural stem cells. A month later he put the rats back into the water maze. The difference couldn't have been more stark. Before the rats didn't learn but now they did, performing statistically the same as rats without Alzheimer's disease. Neural stem cells had "cured" these rats.

But, surprisingly, these stem cells hadn't cured their *brains*. Inside these rats' brains, plaques and tangles remained. "We found absolutely no difference," LaFerla said. "This is unparalleled. This is the first time in our lab—or probably any lab—we've been able to improve Alzheimer's without lowering plaque pathology. Likewise, we had no effect on tangle pathology." And LaFerla saw only a few new neurons. In fact, three of the four markers of Alzheimer's disease were untouched in the cured rats: plaque, tangles, and neurons. But the fourth marker—the number of synapses, or junctions between neurons—bloomed. Injected with neural stem cells, the existing neurons in the hippocampus sprouted tiny connective tendrils, reconnecting the rich lattice of the brain that had been withered by the disease. "That was very interesting, because the best correlate of cognitive decline [due to Alzheimer's disease] is not plaques or tangles but the degree of synaptic loss," LaFerla said.

As LaFerla describes in a 2009 article in the journal *Proceedings of the National Academy of Sciences*, these neural stem cells injected into rat hippocampi secreted a growth factor—in this case something called brain-derived neurotrophic factor, or BDNF—and this growth factor set the brain's repair mechanisms into action, building new synapses between existing neurons. "Essentially the cells were producing fertilizer for the brain," LaFerla says.

Interestingly, when researchers tried to cut out the stem cell middlemen and injected rat brains directly with the growth factor BDNF, they saw similar synaptic growth—but at only *half* the level induced by stem cells.

"We got into this not expecting it to work," LaFerla says. "Now we know stem cells don't need to replace neurons. By implanting stem cells into brains, there is almost a doubling of synaptic density."

This is stem cell treatment at its most promising.

So in addition to growing new tissues, an important feature of stem cells is their ability to act as an ambulance crew, moving from cell to cell looking to heal those in need. This is important: stem cells seem to be able to spot distressed cells, those cells affected by disease. And this feature may allow them not only to deliver their own medicines but to act as delivery systems for next-generation therapies.

At a different University of California campus, UC Davis, researchers are teaching stem cells to deliver genetic therapies to cells affected by one of the cruelest and most lethal neurologic diseases: Huntington's disease.

Your body is made up of between 10 and 100 trillion cells, and in every one of these cells (except for reproductive cells and in some diseases), a chromosome from your father pairs with a chromosome from your mother to create twenty-three tightly bound, double packages that are your body's blueprint. These chromosomes (or actually the genes they contain) tell your body how to build the proteins it needs. When you reproduce, you separate these chromosome pairs, giving twenty-three strands to your child—some that you originally inherited from your father and some that you got from your mother.

In Huntington's disease, there is a defect gene or mutation on the fourth chromosome, and unlike many other genetic diseases, one copy of the faulty gene is enough to create the disease. It's what's called a genetically dominant mutation. If you get a Huntington's chromosome from your mother or your father, you get the disease. It's as terribly, devastatingly clear-cut as that. And so if either of your parents has Huntington's disease, you have exactly a fifty-fifty chance of inheriting the disease yourself. It's a coin flip.

That's the case for twenty-seven-year-old Peggy Down, from (ironically) Huntington Beach, California, who told her story to the California Institute for Regenerative Medicine. When she was nine, her father was diagnosed with Huntington's disease, and since then she has known that she has even odds of carrying the gene herself. She has decided not to undergo the genetic test for the disease, saying, "If I tested positive, I would symptom-search even more than I do now." Because the symptoms of the disease tend to show up in middle life, commonly between ages thirty-five and forty-four, Peggy is on the cusp of the years in which she'll tip one way or the other—a 50 percent chance of being genetically and physically healthy, able to both live her own life and also know that if she chooses to have children, she won't saddle them with the gene. Or in these midlife years, Peggy could tip in the other direction. Huntington's usually starts with a tremor and inevitably progresses into dementia and disability. The disease reduces life expectancy to about twenty years after the first symptoms show up, but the quality of life for many of those years is almost always awful. "I love outdoor activities. I love traveling, reading, talking, walking, eating—I'm very good at eating. I just don't want to give up those things I love most in life: my relationships, my independence," says Peggy.

Just as the coin-flip odds of inheriting Huntington's are simple, the gene that creates it is simple, too. The defect on chromosome number four is a DNA sequence that should be short but instead is long. There are only four little molecules, called nucleotide bases, that write the entire code of the human genome—adenine, thymine, guanine, and cytosine. These four bases of A-T-G-C arranged in long strings tell your body how to make everything it needs, from tissue to hormones. The tiny sequence C-A-G tells your body to make the amino acid glutamine, which does a number of important things in your body. But in Huntington's patients, a section of chromosome 4 is a broken record for C-A-G, telling the patient's body to produce and produce and produce glutamine over and over and over—a length of this chromosome is a repeating string of CAGCAGCAGCAG.

If this C-A-G sequence repeats more than thirty-eight times on chromosome 4, the amino acid glutamine runs amok, creating a new protein called mutant Huntingtin (mHtt) that causes the brain damage of Huntington's disease. Specifically, mHtt eats the spines off a class of brain cells known as spiny neurons. These neurons get their name from the branches that extend from them in every direction, using these branches to entangle and thus communicate with branches from neighboring spiny neurons. Like a lightning-fast and completely accurate kindergarten game of telephone, the signals that control and modulate movement, cognition, and emotion are transmitted from spiny neuron to spiny neuron. Without these spines, neurons stop communicating, and without communicating, movement, cognition, and emotional control decline.

A team led by Jan Nolta, PhD, at the University of California, Davis, taught stem cells to kill mHtt.

After reading the preceding section about Alzheimer's disease, you know that mesenchymal stem cells migrate to the scene of damage and pump out growth factors and other healing agents. In her lab, Nolta, who is stem cell program director at UC Davis, used the natural ability of mesenchymal stem cells to seek out disease. While in the neighborhood, in addition to aiding ailing cells, Nolta hopes MSCs can be taught to step between the faulty gene and its deadly protein. She does this by inserting into the genetic code of the MSCs the ability to interrupt an intermediate step between the faulty Huntington's gene and the creation of the destructive protein mHtt. A quick online video search returns footage of her engineered MSCs in action—they find affected spiny neurons and pump in protective factors, only in this case, along with the protectives, they add the genetically engineered bit that also stops the damage before it's done. The therapy works not only in the petri dish but also in animal studies, drastically decreasing Huntington's symptoms and prolonging survival in mice. Though we'd like to think otherwise, our brains are not so different from those of mice.

Nolta's technology is waiting for a patent before jumping into human trials. "We are hoping to have a real impact in treating this disease," she says.

As for Peggy Down, she says, "Whenever I'm having a rough day, I think about stem cell research. It just gives me hope."

The Huntington's community agrees that for the first time there is a real hope. "This is the best news," said Judy Roberson, president of the Huntington's Disease Society of America, Northern California chapter, in an article on the organization's website. "Families like mine have been waiting for an intervention for Huntington's since the gene was located sixteen years ago. My husband and his brother and thousands of others died waiting for something, anything." Now, thanks to the research at UC Davis, there's real hope.

To provide hope for another neurodegenerative disease, hereditary ataxia, California researchers teamed up with scientists on the other side of the world and then returned to the United States to publish their results in the September 2011 issue of the *Journal of Translational Medicine*. Ataxia describes the umbrella symptoms of loss of balance and coordination, slurred speech, difficulty swallowing, and a handful of unpleasant others that are caused by a range of diseases—but the gist of all these diseases is clear: something has gone wrong at the base of the brain.

For example, in 2003, seventeen-year-old Charlie Ganz of Grand Island, Nebraska, was diagnosed with spinocerebellar ataxia, in which, as the name implies, the brain's cerebellum and very top of the spinal cord decay over time. Because the cerebellum is the home of movement integration, this leads to such symptoms as loss of coordination, which can progress to almost complete loss of muscle control. Different forms of diseases associated with ataxia may result in symptoms ranging from difficulty swallowing, sleep abnormalities, or seizures. In Charlie's case, in addition to coordination difficulties, ataxia stole his sight and was in the process of stealing his speech.

After being a wrestler and playing in his school marching band, Charlie told a Nebraska television program, "I can't read music, and my balance made it hard to march. I love wrestling; I've been doing it since I was six years old, but I just couldn't do it anymore."

After finding their options in the United States limited, Charlie and his family traveled to China for treatment, which used technologies developed by the San Diego biotechnology company Medistem and the Chinese biotechnology company Beike. Into his spine, Charlie received six injections of stem cells derived from donated umbilical cords, followed by rehabilitation therapy.

The published results of the study are striking. The widely used Berg Balance Scale scores patients on fourteen tasks, including things such as standing in different positions with eyes closed, stepping on and off a stool, and standing on one leg. Of the thirty patients enrolled in this study, according to the *Journal of Translational Medicine* article, seventeen patients improved their Berg Balance Scale scores by between 5 and 49 percent. This sounds like a very strong result—that is, until you compare it to the results of the remaining thirteen members of the study, who reported improvement on the Berg Balance Scale *even greater than 50 percent*. The journal reports that the greatest increase was a patient whose score jumped 87.5 percent.

Two months after his treatment, Charlie's mom posted results to a blog that chronicles his journey, writing, "These are some pictures from a vacation to Colorado. Charlie is doing great and made the 1,700-foot ascent. It wasn't easy but he did it!" Photos show Charlie in a tank top, hiking with ski poles for balance on a trail in Winter Park, Colorado. He's handsome and tall, and his arms are noticeably muscled. With a ski lift in the background, Charlie poses on an overlook, back to back with his brother. If you didn't know better, you'd imagine the pair were fit college students on a spring break trip.

Still, a blog update posted on May 24, 2011, two years after his treatment, describes Charlie's difficult journey, including, after initial improvements following treatment, the continued, inexorable march of the disease. His mom describes Charlie, now legally blind, attending community college with the help of a support dog. The picture that accompanies the blog post shows Charlie, who could be a J.Crew model, walking with a black Lab in a mall. His mom writes, "We continue to hold hope for the future and new treatments that are out there on the horizon."

Researchers continue to develop and test stem cell treatments for ataxia. In May 2011, Beike, the Chinese biotechnology company that treated Charlie, started a new iteration of its clinical trial, which you can find at ClinicalTrials.gov under the number NCT01360164.

Like many forms of ataxia and like Huntington's disease, Batten disease is an inherited neurodegenerative genetic condition. But unlike Huntington's, it takes two chromosomes to tango—both a child's mother and father have to give the child a faulty copy of chromosome 16 in order for the child to develop Batten disease. This is known as a recessive genetic disease. On this chromosome 16 is a gene called CLN3, and this gene makes a protein that helps your brain's cleaning crew, the lysosomes. In a healthy brain, these lysosomes float around inside cells, breaking down and throwing waste products like killed and digested viruses and bacteria through the cell wall to the outside, where eventually they're cleansed from your system. Lysosomes are also responsible for cleaning up their own digestive juices, called lipofuscins. Think of these lipofuscins as evil, yellow-brown leprechauns. If these evil leprechaun globs of fat and protein accumulate, they clog and eventually suffocate cells and, critically in this case, neurons.

Because lipofuscin accumulation takes time, babies born with two Batten-defective copies of chromosome 16 are initially healthy. Then, as the leprechauns start to gather in late infancy or early childhood, symptoms may start, including vision and coordination problems and loss of cognitive skills. Later, these symptoms almost always progress to seizures, blindness, and cognitive decline. Eventually, young patients become bedridden and are unable to communicate. Batten disease ultimately is fatal.

Batten disease is one of fifty similar diseases that affect the body's lysosomes, which together affect one in every five thousand children born worldwide.

In a strategy similar to Jan Nolta's of using stem-cell-delivered gene therapy for Huntington's disease, researchers at Weill Cornell Medical College tried using a harmless virus to carry genes into the brains of Batten disease patients. In general, viruses inject genes into a cell that recruit the cell's machinery to make whatever proteins the virus wants—generally more copies of the virus itself. In the Weill Cornell study, researchers made viruses that injected genes into the brain cells of Batten disease patients; these genes replaced the defective gene on chromosome 16, inducing the neurons to manufacture the proteins that lysosomes need in order to do their jobs. This therapy, which has nothing to do with stem cells, successfully slowed the disease's progress.

But it's not a cure. Young Batten disease patients continue to die, only later. Many researchers hope that stem cells will provide an alternative. If using gene therapy to teach a Batten disease patient's brain cells to make the protein it needs doesn't solve the problem, perhaps bombarding the brain with new, healthy cells capable of producing this protein would do the trick.

As of now, that's where this stem cell story of Batten disease ends—with promise. But while clinical trials of stem cells for Batten disease have stalled, similar treatments for Parkinson's disease are pushing forward.

In 2009, University of California, Los Angeles, researcher and Cedars-Sinai Medical Center neurosurgeon Michel Lévesque published the results of a five-year follow-up exam of a Parkinson's disease patient whose brain he had injected with the patient's own concentrated neural stem cells.

Like Huntington's and Batten diseases, Parkinson's is a neurodegenerative disease that results from the death of a specific kind of brain cell. Imagine it this way: in Huntington's disease, a gene gone haywire produces a protein that kills spiny neurons; in Parkinson's disease, the neurons that create dopamine die.

Like the chemical acetylcholine, whose loss is implicated in Alzheimer's disease, the chemical dopamine is a neurotransmitter, meaning that it carries signals from one neuron to another across the junctions called synapses. In order for signals to travel across these specific synapses, your brain needs sufficient dopamine. And in Parkinson's disease, the dopamine-generating cells die in midbrain and thus limit production of the neurotransmitter, leading first to the shaky movements we associate with the disease and later to cognitive problems and often dementia.

As you might know, dopamine is also associated with pleasure. We get dopamine release in the brain naturally through eating and engaging in sexual activity. And we get it artificially through the use of illegal drugs like cocaine and methamphetamines. And so it might seem logical to prescribe regimens of these activities for Parkinson's sufferers. Unfortunately, while eating and cocaine create the impression of more dopamine in the brain, they don't stimulate its production—and in fact drugs like cocaine, morphine, and methamphetamines deplete the brain's dopamine reserves and eventually kill the brain's ability to release dopamine on its own, leading to the very Parkinson's-like symptoms of drug withdrawal.

For example, instead of making more dopamine, the euphoria of cocaine is created both by the drug's ability to increase the secretion of dopamine and by stopping neurons from sucking back up the dopamine they release. By blocking the transport molecule that dopamine needs to get back into neurons, cocaine ensures that more dopamine floats around in the brain, creating pleasure. Of course, this results in less dopamine *inside* the neurons for use next time it's needed.

So, solving the problem of Parkinson's is not as easy as

stimulating dopamine *release*—it's a problem of creating more dopamine itself, and in the right place. The next logical cure is to give Parkinson's patients dopamine in proportion to the amount lost to their disease. Dopamine was already synthesized by George Barger and James Ewens in 1910, so the question raises spontaneously: why not simply augment the dopamine in a Parkinson's patient's brain by daily dopamine injections, the way a diabetic uses insulin? Unfortunately, this strategy is nixed by the size of the dopamine molecule—it's too big to cross the defensive blood-brain barrier and so (to co-opt the Las Vegas catchphrase) dopamine that happens in the circulatory system stays in the circulatory system, where instead of causing euphoria and relief from Parkinson's, this excess dopamine causes such symptoms as nausea, muscle tics, and joint stiffness. You can't inject or ingest dopamine and expect it to affect the brain.

So instead, the common treatment for Parkinson's disease is with drugs that are small enough to cross the blood-brain barrier, which are then manufactured into dopamine once inside the brain. For more than thirty years, the drug levodopa, a dopamine precursor, has been used for just this. But because even levodopa isn't tiny, only 5 to 10 percent of the drug crosses the blood-brain barrier; the excess floats around the circulatory system, wreaking havoc. And the relief of levodopa is short-lived, packing neurons with dopamine that is quickly used up and must be replaced by more of the drug.

Because Parkinson's is a much-studied, visible disease, there are other, newer treatments and combination therapies that lengthen a patient's independence from about eight years if left untreated to fifteen to twenty years with the best treatment (though a 2006 article in the *Journal of Neurology* laments the difficulty in predicting the course of the disease).

This involved and lengthy description is meant to show that better treatments are desperately needed for the estimated 1 percent of people older than sixty and 4 percent of people older than eighty who suffer from Parkinson's disease.

We'll get to Dr. Michel Lévesque's treatment of Parkinson's in a bit. But first let's go to China, where (like many of the overseas treatments described in this book) experimental stem cell therapies have been in wide use for some time. And like stem cell treatments in India or China or Portugal for conditions like stroke and heart disease and spinal cord injury, the anecdotal evidence for stem cell success with Parkinson's disease is compelling enough to at least warrant discussion.

In 2007, fifty-five-year-old UK citizen Janet Whitman traveled to Tiantan Puhua International Hospital in China, where neurosurgeons injected retinal pigment epithelial stem cells cultured from her own cells into her Parkinson's-ravaged brain. When treated, Janet was unable to dress herself, to turn over in bed, or to stand unassisted. She couldn't put on her shoes or turn her neck, and her speech was becoming increasingly slow. In 2007, Janet was becoming defined by what she *couldn't* do. Echoing many patients who resort to costly, unproven overseas treatments, she says, "Those in the West that urge caution for Parkinson's sufferers who consider going to Beijing, with no evidence to say why, simply aren't going through what I have been going through."

Six weeks after treatment, Janet Whitman rode a bicycle.

Likewise, after watching her symptoms progress for five years after being diagnosed with Parkinson's at age fifty-four, American Michelle Dowd followed Janet to China. So did Jason White and Jim Lourdes, both in their midsixties. All reported improvement. For example, Michelle wrote in a blog post that before stem cell therapy, "without heavy medication, I could hardly get dressed, get out of bed, or take a shower on my own. I was a watch keeper. I used to watch the clock all the time. After a time, I stopped swimming and avoided other physical and social activities because I never knew when the medications would wear off." After surgery, Michelle was able to cut her use of the medication Sinemet from 400 mg eight times a day to 200 mg four times a day.

Again, without a carefully controlled clinical trial of this therapy, the benefits remain in the realm of anecdote—did the implantation of retinal stem cells into these Parkinson's patients' brains kick-start their ability to make dopamine, or was it simply the belief borne of this treatment that created these dramatic recoveries? Or maybe there's yet another, unknown mechanism of action?

It's hard to tell. And so it's even harder to tell whether you or your loved ones who are suffering from Parkinson's should follow in these patients' costly, experimental, unproven footsteps. Luckily, researchers are quickly straightening the long and winding road of stem cell treatment for Parkinson's disease.

By 1999, fifty-seven-year-old Ron Jones had tried everything American medicine had to offer, including 600 mg of daily levodopa and deep brain stimulation of his left thalamus to control his tremors. In testimony before the United States Senate Commerce Subcommittee on Science, Technology, and Space, Ron told chairman Sam Brownback and the other members, "I suffered extreme shaking of the right side of my body, stiffness in my gait and movements. . . . My disability prevented me from using my right arm." He had progressed to stage four on the widely used Hoehn and Yahr scale, defined as "severe disability but still able to walk or stand unassisted." This is the second-to-last stage of the disease.

But due in part to a high degree of physical fitness outside

Parkinson's disease, UCLA's Dr. Lévesque felt Ron was a good candidate for his FDA-approved clinical trial. It was during implantation of Ron's electrical deep-brain stimulating device that Lévesque sampled 90 cubic millimeters of Ron's prefrontal cortical and subcortical brain regions, removing a cube about half the size of playing dice.

Lévesque then treated this removed brain tissue in the lab with a complex procedure over the course of six months, cutting it into tiny pieces, placing it in a solution, spinning it in a centrifuge to separate the stem cells, and then growing the stem cells in the presence of a growth factor to coax them into becoming mature dopamine neurons. After six months, he split the sample into vials and tested the results. Yes, the vials contained mature dopamine neurons; yes, when tested, these new neurons produced dopamine; and yes, the samples had remained sterile.

And then Lévesque injected these carefully crafted mature dopamine neurons back into the part of Ron's brain where dopamine would normally be released—6 million dopaminergic neurons in all, of which lab studies predicted around 93,000 would survive in Ron's brain (compared to an estimated 250,000 dopaminergic neurons in a hemisphere of the healthy substantia nigra—the region of the brain affected by Parkinson's). Before and after his operation, Ron underwent pretty much every neurological and imaging test you can imagine, hoping to define with pinpoint accuracy exactly what the treatment had or hadn't done.

And here is what happened.

"Soon after having the cells injected, my Parkinson's symptoms began to improve. My trembling grew less and less, until to all appearances it was gone, only slightly reappearing if I became upset. Dr. Lévesque had me tested by a neurologist, who said he wouldn't have known I had Parkinson's if he had met me on the street. I was once again able to use my right hand and arm normally, enjoying activities that I given up hope of ever doing," he told the US Senate subcommittee.

Lévesque's clinical follow-up confirms Ron's description. Before treatment, Ron's score on the Unified Parkinson's Disease Rating Scale was 37 of a possible 100, and after treatment, his score jumped to 70. This was without medication! After treatment, when taking medication, Ron scored a full 100 points on this scale—the same score as a person without the disease. Nine months after treatment, his tremor that had before been moderately controlled by deep brain stimulation was gone, even without medication and without stimulation.

Then, Ron told the Senate committee, "last year [2003], after four years of being virtually symptom-free, my Parkinson's symptoms began reappearing in my body's left side." At forty-eight months after treatment, he again started to sink into his disease. And at five years posttreatment, at sixty-two years old, Ron was back almost exactly where he had been before Lévesque injected his brain with neural stem cells. But his remission was unprecedented—after progressing to stage-four Parkinson's disease, Ron had spent four years almost completely symptom free.

"I have no doubt that because of this treatment I've enjoyed five years of quality life that I feared had passed me by," Ron said. Maybe you've heard the cliché "a new lease on life." Lévesque's treatment of Ron Jones was literally a five-year lease.

"Because of my improvements through Dr. Lévesque's treatment, I've been able to indulge in my passion for big-game photography these past five years," Ron told the Senate committee. "While on safari in 2001 I scrambled up a tree to avoid being run over by a rhino. I swam in the South Atlantic with great white sharks. Two weeks ago I returned from Africa after photographing cheetahs and leopards in the wild. Here are a few examples of the pictures I took." He then displayed wildlife shots for the senators. "They represent memories and experiences I feel I have Dr. Lévesque to thank for. I came here to offer him my sincere gratitude and to offer others with Parkinson's a concrete reason for hope."

For sufferers of Alzheimer's, Huntington's, Batten, and Parkinson's diseases, stem cell treatments offer more than hope. In these few preliminary trials, they offer good years of life. Perhaps soon they'll offer a cure.

Chapter 8

Tendons, Ligaments, Cartilage, and Bone

Bartolo Colón knows how to make a baseball glove from a milk carton and a ball from tightly wound rags. That's because Bartolo grew up in the three-thousand-person town of Altamira in the Dominican Republic, in a house with no electricity, running water, or indoor plumbing. With his brothers and sister, the young Bartolo frequently joined his father in the bean fields, working very hard every day. He built a pitching arm by throwing rocks to knock coconuts from trees.

In 2005, Bartolo went 21–8 for the Anaheim Angels en route to a 3.48 ERA and the American League Cy Young Award. The Angels made the playoffs that year, and in the division series they faced the New York Yankees. After struggling in the postseason opener, Bartolo took the mound for game five, with the best-of-five series tied at two apiece. The winner of game five would face the Chicago White Sox in the American League Championship Series.

Then in the second inning, after throwing what looked like just another 96+ mph pitch, Bartolo grabbed his right shoulder and walked off the mound. The Angels won the game and the series, but Bartolo didn't pitch in the ALC series against the

White Sox. And then, even after a winter of aggressive rehabil-itation therapy, he went 1–5 in ten starts with a 5.11 ERA at the beginning of the 2006 season—mediocre stats at best. Finally, with persistent soreness in his right shoulder, Bartolo had an MRI, and the injury was obvious: the best pitcher in the Ameri-can League had torn his rotator cuff.

It's a tricky injury—instead of just a hinge like an elbow or a knee, the shoulder spins 360 degrees and is strapped together with a complex mat of muscles and tendons. In Bartolo's rotator cuff injury, he had torn one of these tendons and likely irritated much of the surrounding tissues, too. Bartolo spent four years on and off the disabled list, in and out of Major League Base-ball, fighting the injury.

Colón's creaky shoulder kept him out of the 2010 season en-tirely, and it looked like the aging pitcher's career was over. What few people knew at the time was that in April 2010, he visited Florida doctor Joseph Purita. Purita harvested stem cells from Bartolo's skin and fat, purified them, and injected them into the big right-hander's chronically injured shoulder. The procedure was done in Colón's native Dominican Republic.

Colón's stem cell treatment was scrutinized by Major League Baseball because of concern that human growth hormone, which is banned by MLB, was involved. Dr. Purita had used HGH on other patients but denied using it on Colón, and ulti-mately the MLB investigation determined there was no wrong-doing.

In 2011, the New York Yankees gave Bartolo a tryout, invit-ing him to their preseason training camp to compete for a spot in the rotation. He made the team as a replacement, and when pitcher Phil Hughes was injured, Bartolo took his place. On May 30, 2011, he threw a four-hit complete game shutout. In 2012, he signed on with the Oakland Athletics and in one game threw thirty-eight consecutive pitches for strikes. The one piece of hardware Bartolo was lacking in his long career was a World Series ring. In 2012, years after most managers and fans wrote him off as injured and over-the-hill, Bartolo was back in the game, throwing 95 mph fastballs in pursuit of this ring.

Since then, Colón tested positive for a synthetic form of testosterone and was suspended by Major League Baseball in August of 2012. There's no evidence that Colón used steroids during his stem cell treatment or recovery, although testosterone is said to speed muscle healing so it may have helped the treatment's effectiveness. Still, steroid users have not had much success healing torn rotator cuffs without stem cells, and in any case, unless you play professional or collegiate sports, adding testosterone to a stem cell treatment isn't prohibited.

Despite tipping the scales at 265 pounds, Bartolo Colón is a pitching thoroughbred, with an arm that continues to put a two-seam fastball over the plate at 95 mph as a thirty-nine-year-old. The stem cell technique that brought him back to this form was pioneered in another kind of thoroughbred. Roger Smith, a professor at the Royal Veterinary College and veterinarian with the British bioscience firm VetCell, published the results of his stem cell treatment of racehorses in the *British Journal of Sports Medicine* under the title "Harnessing the Stem Cell for the Treatment of Tendon Injuries: Heralding a New Dawn?" In the paper, Smith describes the injuries, treatment, and recoveries of 581 racehorses.

The career of a thoroughbred racehorse is a short one to begin with, with horses tending to retire at about four or five years old. In that time, a horse will make a rough average of only about twenty starts. Of the 581 horses treated with Smith's stem cell therapy, exactly 74.4 percent returned to racing after their injuries. But even more impressive might be the fact that 55 of these horses then went on to run ten or more races. Imagining that more than half of these horses' injuries occurred more than halfway through the natural course of their careers and that treatment was followed by almost a year of careful rehabilitation, the ability to run ten or more starts after a tendon injury almost necessarily means that these fifty-five horses ran past the age they would have retired had they not been injured.

Right now, because stem cell treatment for tendon injuries isn't approved by the FDA, patients who want the procedure have to search for clinics and then pay the expense out-of-pocket. But that's likely to change soon. VetCell has a sister company called MedCell, which in 2011 received approval for a human clinical trial based on well-performed initial research on animal (horse) models. Can humans expect the same 80 percent success rate of thoroughbred horses? Twenty-four lucky test patients with Achilles tendonitis will find out.

Even in the rest of us who don't happen to be Cy Young Award–winning pitchers (or endurance racehorses), the years grind down our bodies—cartilage is pounded flat, small tweaks and tears accumulate, and bone thins. And now, for each of these problems, there are developing stem cell cures.

For example, on July 1, 2011, then-incumbent governor of Texas and 2012 presidential candidate Rick Perry received experimental stem cell surgery in hopes of fixing a bad back. Much like the treatments for Bartolo Colón and the racehorses, doctors harvested some of Perry's fat cells, cultured and concentrated the stem cells from this tissue, and then injected the stem cells back into his spine and bloodstream. Perry hoped the infusion of adult mesenchymal stem cells would help heal the bones of his spine after they were fused during the surgery.

While Perry reports being pleased with the outcome, the FDA has made it clear that this spinal fusion surgery is in need of clinical trial success to ensure it becomes standard of care. Current methods of helping bone heal after spinal fusion include implanting bone tissue from the patient's hip or from a cadaver to encourage bone regrowth. Doctors have also studied the use of protein-based bone growth factors, but a recent review in the *Spine Journal* by its editor, an orthopedic surgeon at Stanford, showed that these bone growth factors can carry with them an increased chance of male sterility, urinary problems, infection, bone and nerve injuries, and increased cancer risk.

In another study, UC Davis researchers found that adequate spinal fusion failed to occur in 25 percent of tested patients, and persistent pain occurred in up to 60 percent of these patients with fusion failure, often necessitating additional surgery.

"A lack of effective new bone growth after spine fusion surgery can be a significant problem, especially in surgeries involving multiple spinal segments," said Rudolph Schrot, co-principal investigator of the UC Davis study.

So, medicine's question is how to make the bone heal together, ensuring the vertebrae fuse and stay fused. Could stem cells make the mortar between these two bones? If so, the addition of stem cells to the procedure could help the estimated 230,000 Americans who are currently candidates for spinal fusion surgery.

"For the past fifty years, bone-marrow-derived stem cells have been used to rebuild patients' blood-forming systems. We know that subsets of stem cells from the marrow also can robustly build bone. Their use now to promote vertebral fusion is a new and extremely promising area of clinical study," said Jan Nolta, director of the UC Davis Institute for Regenerative Cures.

While it's wonderful that stem cells added to spinal fusion surgery will very likely lower the rate of post-op complications, even better is that within five years, stem cells should offer an alternative to spinal fusion altogether. In degenerative disc disease, the padding of these discs wears down, leaving the bones of the spinal column to grate against each other. It's a chronic, painful condition that usually starts with lower back pain and can migrate into the hips, legs, and even upward into the neck, where this chronic pain can result in headaches and even, eventually, loss of cognitive function. Literally, the pain of degenerative disc disease can drive sufferers crazy. But biomedical engineer Larry Bonassar of Cornell University is only a few steps away from curing the bad back of degenerative disc disease with the implant of spinal discs grown from a patient's own stem cells.

It's tricky. "The spinal disc is nonvascularized," Bonassar says, "so you can't just use tissue growth strategies. You have to make something new. Plus it's kind of a dense tissue that's hard to migrate through." In other words, blood vessels don't invade the spinal disc tissue, and unlike tendon repair, in which you can inject stem cells and let them do their work, the spinal disc is too dense to allow stem cells to move around in order to provide the kind of rescue and repair they do in other tissues.

So, instead of tissue repair, Bonassar works with tissue replacement.

In July 2011, Bonassar, along with Weill Cornell Medical Center neurosurgeon Roger Härtl, published results of their spinal disc engineering project in the highly respected journal *Proceedings of the National Academy of Sciences*. In short, Bonassar and Härtl built a new disc.

First, similar to procedures we've seen elsewhere in this book, Bonassar seeded stem cells onto a collagen model. But contrary to the popular image of a simple, round cushion, a spinal disc actually looks more like a donut with a membrane stretched across the hole in its middle. The cake of the donut cups the outside of the bony spinal column, and the inner jelly filling of the donut provides the majority of the cushioning between vertebrae. So in addition to a collagen model that provided the structure for the donut itself, Bonassar used a hydrogel called alginate to span the hole in the donut's center.

And then, instead of simply seeding the lattice with bone-marrow-derived stem cells, Bonassar says, "Our twist on this is that we incorporate it with technology we've invented for tissue injection molding so that when it comes out of the mold, we have a living implant." Basically, this tissue injection is like the industrial process of injection molding in which plastic is injected into a mold, where it cools—only in this case, instead of plastic into a mold, Bonassar injected stem cells into a collagen architecture, helping them stay compressed into the durable shape of a spinal disc.

Once Bonassar engineered a spinal disc, he handed the project to neurosurgeon Härtl. Bonassar describes the results: "We removed an intact disc from a rat, replaced it with the engineered disc, and for the duration of the rat's natural life, the disc functioned perfectly." In fact, because the rat's body recognized the disc's stem cells and so healed the disc into its spinal architecture, "the mechanical properties only got better with time," Bonassar says. As cells continued to grow in and around the implanted disc, its function improved (rather than degraded, as do all current spinal disc replacements made of bone, metal, or plastic). Over rats' lives, the discs retained 80 to 90 percent of their height.

Because Cornell University has one of the top veterinary schools in the country, Bonassar imagines soon being able to move the technology into larger animals, including dogs and maybe horses. Human application is still a couple years out, but Bonassar's sleight-of-hand switch of a rat's spinal disc for one engineered from stem cells puts the end of suffering from degenerative disc disease firmly within the inevitable future.

In the further future, biotechnology researchers like Bonassar imagine working with induced pluripotent stem cells (adult stem cells genetically reprogrammed to an embryonic-like state) to "turn it into an off-the-shelf kind of product," he says. Another option gaining steam is work by the biotechnology company NeoStem with very small embryonic-like cells (VSELs)—the body's naturally pluripotent stem cells—to build similar discs from scratch, but without the problems of potential rejection and tumor formation currently faced by induced pluripotent cells.

And Bonassar points to the work of researchers led by Charlie Archer, professor at Cardiff University's School of Biosciences, who recently found stem cells that are specialized to create cartilage. "Cartilage isn't limited to the material of spinal discs," Bonassar says. "In fact, cartilage is a family of tissues. Maybe it's made up of 10,000 proteins, and all cartilage shares 9,500 of these proteins, but maybe 500 of the proteins in knee cartilage are different than the proteins in spinal disc cartilage." In Bonassar's opinion, finding stem cells that are specialized to create certain tissues, even down to the difference between knee and spinal disc cartilage, allows less fiddling by scientists to ensure these stem cells, in fact, create the right tissues.

"If you start with embryonic stem cells or even induced pluripotent stem cells, you have to program all ten thousand proteins," says Bonassar. By finding adult stem cells that are specialized to the tissue they're supposed to create, all scientists may have to do is inject them (in the case of Bartolo Colón's rotator cuff surgery) or sculpt them (in the case of Bonassar's spinal discs).

"If all goes well, if the tech shows the same legs as it did in rats, we're talking about an order of five years for people," says Bonassar.

A similar fast track from animals to humans is likely in the case of the treatment for nine-year-old golden retriever Hunter, who lives with his owners, Frank and Linda Riha, in Burbank, California. Like many aging large purebred dogs, Hunter has hip dysplasia, in which a slight malformation of the hip socket results in looseness, which in turn over time causes abnormal wear and tear in the joint and eventually arthritis.

The ABC news program *Nightline* profiled Hunter and quoted Linda describing the friendly golden retriever as "a celebrity on our street" and saying about his hip dysplasia that "his leg, it's almost like it's lifeless and it'll drift back." The Golden Retriever Club of America reports that between 20 and 30 percent of adult golden retrievers have dysplastic hips. Joint supplements like glucosamine show some benefits, and nonsteroidal anti-inflammatories like carprofen (like ibuprofen for dogs) can both reduce swelling and ease pain. But the only "cure" for advanced hip dysplasia is surgery—either removing and reshaping the head of the femur or a total hip replacement. Both these surgical options are rather short-lasting and expensive, costing upward of $10,000 for a replacement.

Still, *Nightline* quoted Linda as saying, "He's just special. He's just a good boy and I get emotional, but it's 'cause I love him so much." And so the couple was ready to explore the expensive and imperfect fix of a hip replacement. That is, until their doctor offered an alternative. For about $2,500 they could try stem cell therapy.

Hunter's owners chose stem cells, and vets harvested about 30 grams of Hunter's body fat (which may have contributed to the slightly chubby Hunter's dysplasia pain in the first place). The fat was then whisked off to the nearby lab of the biotechnology company Vet-Stem in San Diego, which broke up the fat cells and spun them in a centrifuge to separate the stem cells.

Twenty-four hours later, Hunter's vet injected this concentrated mixture of stem cells into the good old retriever's arthritic hip.

Two weeks later, Frank told ABC, "He jumped up on the bed, which is almost three feet tall, and he hasn't done that in quite a few months, and we kind of freaked out because he's supposed to stay quiet, but he was right up there and ready to go."

Vet-Stem reports similar results with 70 percent of its animal patients, including the racehorse Be a Bono, who returned from his stem cell therapy to win $1.25 million in prize money.

And remember when we talked about knee cartilage? Well, researchers at Wake Forest are nearing the ability to grow a new meniscus.

When you picture the bones that cross behind a skull on a pirate flag, you picture something very much like the human tibia, with its two knobby platforms on the top, or the human femur, with two knobs on the bottom. If these knobs sat directly on top of each other, walking would be a very painful experience, punctuated by loud bone-on-bone grinding. Your ability to walk without your tibia rubbing against your femur is due to a tough piece of cartilage known as your meniscus, which is shaped like a figure eight, into which the knobs of the tibia and femur sit. Tears in the meniscus are the most common cause of knee surgery.

A little tear can feel like a click or an ache and is easy to fix—arthroscopic surgery can cut out the torn tissue and smooth the rest. This is what's actually done when you hear that an athlete had his or her knee "scoped." It sounds like a routine procedure, and in most cases it is, but enough scoping over enough time (or a worse injury) can result in an irreparable meniscus. In this case, the best surgical option is to switch the damaged meniscus for a replacement, usually taken from a cadaver.

Unfortunately, the body has the bad habit of keeping a cadaver meniscus at arm's length—while the body doesn't usually reject the replacement like it might a mismatched donor organ, it tends not to embrace donor menisci either. A patient's cells usually don't grow into the central part of cadaver menisci, meaning that these implants rarely function as well or last as long as the original cartilage. It's an imperfect fix.

Like Cornell bioengineer Larry Bonassar's spinal disc, researchers at Wake Forest, including Julie Steen, Cristin Ferguson, and Mark Van Dyke, are working to implant patients' stem cells into bio-lattices shaped like their own menisci. These stem cell transplants work in mice and are working their way toward humans.

The day can't come soon enough for Lyle Buchanan, who told his story to the management team at NeoStem when he went to the company to bank his stem cells in anticipation of future stem cell treatments. "About two and a half years ago," he explained, "I woke up one morning, and I was in tremendous pain, just like instantaneous, in my knees." Lyle was diagnosed with degenerative osteoarthritis. "My knees were almost bone on bone, and I needed a double knee replacement . . . already," he said. "Two and a half years ago I was with my son in Vermont snowboarding. And just to wake up like that and be completely debilitated was amazing."

Lyle went through two orthopedic surgeries in hopes of correcting the problem. "No success," he says. "The pain is unbearable. Completely unbearable."

At fifty-one years old, Lyle doesn't want to wait for Wake Forest's stem cell meniscus, which should be ready for prime time around 2020. Instead, he and others like him can transplant stem cells into damaged cartilage instead of transplanting the entire cartilage itself. Pioneered by Dr. Christopher Centeno of the Centeno-Schultz Clinic in Broomfield, Colorado, harvesting, concentrating, and then injecting a patient's stem cells into damaged cartilage is showing promising results. For one example among many, in 2010 after a failed meniscus repair surgery, two-time Super Bowl Champion defensive end Jarvis Green was cut by the Denver Broncos, where he was playing as a free agent. Jarvis turned to Centeno's Regenexx technology as a treatment of last hope. Where surgery and rehab failed, Regenexx succeeded, and before the 2011 season Jarvis was signed by the Houston Texans. (For more information on Dr. Centeno and his Regenexx procedure, see chapter 11.)

In another futuristic treatment, again at Wake Forest, researchers are growing stem-cell-seeded muscles on long ropes of collagen, which are then "exercised" in a computer-controlled machine that stretches and flexes the tissue as it grows. According to the Wake Forest School of Medicine website, this seeding and stretching "allows the cells to align in one direction, fuse to form muscle bundles, and function like normal muscle."

And especially for combat veterans, Wake Forest hopes to replace lost ears with implants seeded with patients' own cartilage stem cells. This, they hope, will reduce the common problems of infection and "protrusion from the skin" of current, ear-shaped prosthetics.

As you've noticed, this is not a history book. It's a book about the present and future, and as you're reading this, the story is being written just minutes, weeks, and months ahead of you. Right now millions of people who suffer with degenerative disc disease are waiting for Larry Bonassar's replacement spinal disc to make its way from mice to men. But also right now, hundreds of horses and dogs are up and running after successful, proven stem cell treatments. And despite his subsequent suspension for steroid use after his stem cell therapy, pitcher Bartolo Colón was able to go back on the mound because of the stem cell treatment of his torn rotator cuff.

Chapter 9

ALS: Lou Gehrig's Disease

"Today I consider myself the luckiest man on the face of the earth," Lou Gehrig told 61,808 fans at Yankee Stadium on July 4, 1939. Two years later, and exactly sixteen years to the day after replacing Wally Pip as the Yankee's first baseman, Gehrig died at his home in the Riverdale neighborhood of the Bronx.

From then on, amyotrophic lateral sclerosis, or ALS, has been known as Lou Gehrig's disease. Commonly, patients diagnosed with Lou Gehrig's disease die two to five years after their diagnosis, and 90 percent die by year six, usually of respiratory complications and pneumonia born of the shutdown of motor neurons that drive the muscles of breathing.

Hank Maddie, founding director of Family Focus Christian Counseling in El Cajon, California, tells about his first symptoms: "We have a beautiful home that sits on the side of a very steep cliff," he told an audience of CIRM doctors and researchers, "and I remember first using a hoe as I'm going up the hill and, yes, taking care of weeds but also using it as a crutch, not even realizing why."

He described the disease progressing from the muscles of his legs into his chest, back, arms, and hands: "As a hobby I used to make jewelry for my wife. My daughter asked for a simple thing to be made, and I can't do it. My hands don't work to make a simple piece of jewelry."

The motor neurons that are the target of ALS extend down from the brain to other motor neurons in the spinal cord. From there, nerve fibers called axons extend out to touch and control muscles in every part of the body, like the strings of a marionette that stretch down from the control rod to the doll's feet and hands. The symptoms of ALS occur when these strings are disconnected—when motor neurons in the brain and spinal cord wither and die. When muscles no longer receive signals from nerves, they too wither and waste away.

As the muscles of the diaphragm and rib cage weaken, so, too, does their ability to expand the chest and draw air into the lungs. Most victims of ALS die of this respiratory failure.

While ALS ravages the body, it cruelly leaves the mind intact. Almost all patients retain memory, personality, and cognition, able to watch with absolute understanding the machinery of their muscles shut down and their bodies atrophy before their very eyes.

There is no cure. In fact, despite five thousand cases diagnosed in the United States every year and a nearly 150-year history of recognition, there is exactly one drug approved by the FDA to treat Lou Gehrig's disease—riluzole, which works to lengthen the time ALS patients spend without needing a mechanical ventilator and extends life expectancy by a couple months.

How is it possible in the twenty-first century that we can do little more than watch over the course of years as motor neurons lose their function? How is it possible that after 150 years, all we can do is manage such symptoms of ALS as muscle cramps, excess saliva, pain, depression, and sleep problems while leaving the disease itself untouched? How is it possible that the best treatment for ALS is physical therapy, occupational therapy, assistive technology, and eventually palliative care administered in a hospice facility?

In a disease that seems as simple as motor neurons releasing their grip, and with millions of dollars spent every year on research, it is surprising that the sum of today's medical science does little more than help ALS patients die with some comfort, rather than help them live.

"As a counselor, as a Christian, I believe your mind impacts what happens in your body," Hank said. "I love the fact that God says he gives us the grace for today. He doesn't talk about next week."

And so it's in today that Hank chooses to live.

"A year and a half ago, a friend of mine took me over to a place in La Jolla called the glider port and he assisted in pushing me off the cliff. I went tandem and flew up in the air for about forty-five minutes . . . I am going to enjoy today because later on things will be worse. This disease is a process, and for me it's called surrender," he said.

But just as Hank is learning to surrender, doctors are learning to fight. But one of the most difficult questions with ALS is what, exactly, to fight *against*? Discovering and developing new drug treatments typically relies on the ability to pinpoint a specific gene or cellular process that has gone wrong in a disease—a target. Once you find the target that causes the disease, you can work to correct it. In 1991, researchers found a gene responsible for familial ALS, a heritable version of the disease that accounts for about 5 percent of cases. In healthy people, the gene SOD1 makes an enzyme that protects the body against toxic waste products. But in this subpopulation of heritable ALS patients, a mutated SOD1 leaves the body unable to protect itself from a type of "free radical," which both sounds and acts like a violent political terrorist. These unprotected neurons are poisoned and die.

Recently, researchers discovered two other genes in addition to SOD1 that are possible culprits of familial ALS. Now the question is, which is the cause? And like other heritable diseases, which, when reversed, could provide the cure?

To study this question, researchers used something called knockout mice. These are mice in which certain genes have been turned off—in this case, one or two or three of the genes associated with familial ALS (notice the power of these animal models for research). And this is unique: in mice that were engineered to develop ALS, when researchers turned off these three genes in the motor neurons themselves, the pace of the disease was unchanged. But when they turned off these genes in the cells *surrounding* these motor neurons, ALS mice lived twice as long. In familial ALS, it seems it's not that motor neurons die so much as that their neighbors kill them, thereby driving the progress of symptoms. Or if the neighbors don't exactly kill neurons, at least they're not fulfilling their duties to nourish and sustain them.

But what if researchers could replace these toxic neighbors with friendly ones? That is exactly the strategy of Life Technologies of Carlsbad, California, which is growing stem cells that can generate new, friendly astrocytes (cellular neighbors) to replace the toxic ones in ALS patients. Animal trials are promising, and human trials are expected to start in the next four years.

And while the quest to engineer stem cells that become more effective astrocytes is underway, stem cells are also being used to create better ALS models. Remember that the only existing model of ALS depends on artificially mutating the genes that cause the heritable form of the disease in mice—the form that accounts for only 5 percent of cases. Well, Dr. Eva Feldman, the Russell N. DeJong Professor of Neurology at the University of Michigan, used induced pluripotent stem (iPS) cells to finally create a model of the disease that represents the other 95 percent.

She did this by sampling skin from ALS patients and then scrubbing clean the DNA blueprint that makes these cells become skin, returning the cells to their pluripotent state. So instead of churning out only skin cells, these newly created stem cells become capable of creating many tissue types. Then Feldman coaxes these iPS cells into creating motor neurons—the nerve cells that degenerate in ALS patients. Sure enough, these harvested and reprogrammed motor neuron cells develop the disease. What's different between these ALS motor neurons and another person's healthy motor neurons? This model created with induced pluripotent stem cells should help Feldman and other researchers discover the answer, giving doctors a target for treatment.

In the meantime, it seems as if stem cells should be useful on the therapeutic side. Irrespective of the genetic targets of ALS that may emerge from Feldman's study of induced pluripotent stem cell lines from ALS patients, couldn't you flip the use of iPS cells, injecting healthy ones into patients and letting them work their magic? It seems like a good idea, but it's not. Currently, when released to roam free-range through the body, iPS cells tend to do inconvenient things like create tumors. Also, they may retain a bit of "memory" of the cells they came from, sprinkling remnants of the diseased tissue amid the new tissue. And in certain cases, the body may recognize iPS cells as foreign and attack them.

But the promise remains: if not iPS cells, then maybe another kind of stem cell? One logical choice is NeoStem's work with very small embryonic-like stem cells (VSELs), which have iPS-like pluripotency, but because they can be harvested directly from a patient's body, they don't carry the same problems of rejection and tumor formation. Their use for ALS is still years off, but the hope is that VSELs could replace iPS cells as the pluripotent cell of choice for use with patients.

But while these technologies are still a ways off, autologous, adult stem cells as a treatment for ALS are already in clinical trials, specifically at the Mayo Clinic and at Israel's Hadassah Medical Center in Jerusalem.

In fact, the trial underway in Jerusalem is similar to Life Technologies' futuristic strategy of using stem cells to create healthy astrocytes, but with one important difference. The Israeli researchers don't ask stem cells to make new astrocytes but only to make the beneficial proteins these astrocytes create in healthy people. Here's how it works: First they harvest an adult ALS patient's stem cells from his bone marrow, and then in the lab they culture these cells in a way that encourages them to produce "neurotrophic factors" that support neuron health. After inducing these mesenchymal stem cells to produce these protective factors, these stem cells are injected back into the patient they came from. In twelve patients with early-stage ALS, these stem cells were injected into their biceps and triceps. In twelve patients with more advanced ALS, these cells were injected through a lumbar puncture into their lower backs. As with most clinical trials, this first test, begun in June 2011, was designed mostly to prove the therapy's safety.

In July 2011, the *MDA/ALS Newsmagazine* reported that the biotechnology company BrainStorm was in early-stage planning to bring the Israeli trial to the United States, specifically to Massachusetts General Hospital in Boston and to the University of Massachusetts Medical School in Worcester.

Dr. Eva Feldman said of the current climate of ALS research, "With improvements in the understanding of the causes of ALS, along with the continued development of stem cell therapies, we are poised for the first time to give hope to patients suffering from this devastating and incurable disease, and numerous other neurological conditions as well."

This hope likely won't turn into practice soon enough to help Hank Maddie, the sixty-four-year-old Christian counselor, but he believes "the research is going to help thousands of people down the road, and I think that's wonderful."

Chapter 10

Multiple Sclerosis and Neuromyelitis Optica

"A lot of ladies in the lab have a lot of lip gloss at the Mayo Clinic," cosmetics mogul Victoria Jackson told a group of doctors and researchers from the California Institute for Regenerative Medicine. "I didn't graduate high school, didn't go to college; I spent a lot of time in a lab making lip gloss and beauty products. But when my sixteen-year-old daughter Emma was diagnosed with neuromyelitis optica, a rare disease closely related to multiple sclerosis, I realized I had to go from mascara to medicine."

Multiple sclerosis (MS) and its cousin neuromyelitis optica (NMO) result in the loss of the fatty sheath that insulates neurons. Imagine you're using an electric weed whacker: if the extension cord's plastic and rubber coating has a hole, the electricity leaks out (okay, not exactly, but you get the drift). This is what happens in the brains and spinal cords of patients with MS or NMO.

"One day my daughter said she was suffering from an eyeball headache, and over the next couple days, she started to lose her vision," said Victoria. "The eye doctor said something was going on with her optic nerve. He ordered a test for NMO."

In fact, NMO acts quickly and brutally. One of the doctors told Victoria that she could have four more years with her daughter, and there would be a good chance the young girl would be blind and paralyzed. She and her husband were devastated.

Candace Coffee, who was diagnosed with the disease while doing volunteer work in Tibet, describes symptoms including "temporary bouts of blindness, paralysis, your body's buzzing with electricity, one side of your body is burning, the other side is freezing. It sounds like a science-fiction disease—your legs don't feel, your eyes don't see; everything is placed on hold until you can get your body in control again. Our bodies are surprisingly resilient, but the human spirit takes a really solid beating."

So, Victoria did what any mom who had sold half a billion dollars' worth of cosmetics on infomercials would do—she found the world's top experts on NMO, sat them in a room, and offered to write a check for whatever they needed to cure the disease. But rather than relegate herself to an uninvolved funding source, "it became very apparent to me very quickly that I wouldn't have to just be Mom on a mission, but I'd have to become Dr. Mom." And so in addition to writing checks, Victoria became an expert on NMO, managing every aspect of the top-notch research and treatment team she had assembled.

A few months after her diagnosis, Emma had her first spinal attack. Around the long, wirelike length of a nerve fiber (called the axon) that conducts electrical signals is a fatty layer made out of myelin that insulates it. In multiple sclerosis and neuromyelitis optica, a patient's own immune system turns on this myelin sheath, attacking it as if it were an invading virus and eating away at this fatty insulation until axons leak electricity. Like pouring water into a leaky pipe, electrical signals that travel down an axon without its myelin coat lose power as they travel, becoming weaker. In neuromyelitis optica, the nerves connecting the eyes to the brain are the first targets. In Emma, the immune system had progressed to its secondary target: the nerves of the spinal cord.

During her attack, Emma was nearly paralyzed. Afterward, she recovered. NMO, like some forms of multiple sclerosis, is a disease that comes in clusters of attacks followed by unpredictable remission. The question was: when would Emma's next attack occur? While powerful drugs kept her malfunctioning immune system in check, her mom sprinted for the cure.

At the same time, researchers working on NMO's better-known cousin, multiple sclerosis, were getting closer to a cure. In MS, "abnormal inflammation leads to nervous system damage," says Dr. Jeffrey Cohen, neurologist at the Mellen Center for Multiple Sclerosis Treatment and Research in the Cleveland Clinic. "And in the later stages of the disease, this nervous damage becomes a degenerative process." In other words, there are two challenges in treating MS—stopping the damage of the immune system's inflammatory response and repairing any damage that's been done.

Stem cells are already being used to stop the damage, and Cohen is running a first-of-its-kind clinical trial to explore using stem cells for the repair as well.

Let's take the first thing first—stopping the damage of an MS patient's immune system run amok. And for that we have to briefly leave Victoria Jackson and her daughter Emma, leave Cohen and the Cleveland Clinic, and even leave the twenty-first century and head west to Northwestern University in Chicago. It was at Northwestern in 1996 that Dr. Richard Burt, chief of immunotherapy for autoimmune diseases at Northwestern University's Feinberg School of Medicine, and his colleagues first tried a logical fix: if a faulty immune system attacks myelin and causes multiple sclerosis, why not replace the immune system with a new one that doesn't? This immune system switch is tricky, but it's been the common treatment for leukemia since 1968 (more on this in chapter 14 on cancer).

This is a bone marrow transplant. Because stem cells in bone marrow create the components of the immune system, obliterating a patient's marrow with chemotherapy and radiation and then replacing it with the marrow of a matched donor should create a new, ideally less self-destructive immune system.

Richard Burt wrote about the increasing use of bone marrow transplantation as a treatment for MS in a 2003 issue of the journal *Bone Marrow Transplantation*. His numbers are impressive, but maybe more telling is the experience of one of his patients, Nick Blanchard, who posted a description of his disease and treatment to Dr. Burt's website (http://www.stemcell-immunotherapy.org) on June 6, 2010, nearly seven years after his stem cell treatment for multiple sclerosis.

Nick wrote that "after experiencing bouts of numbness in my legs while vacationing in Las Vegas...I knew something was wrong and made an appointment to see my doctor. Referred to a neurologist, I underwent a MRI and spinal tap. The result was a diagnosis in May of 1995 of multiple sclerosis."

A monthly IV drip of the drug steroid Solu-Medrol generally kept Nick in remission, minus four relapses in June 1995, July 1996, September 2000, and May 2011, which required extended hospital stays. As his MS progressed he added medications, including weekly injections of Avonex, a type of interferon, which he gave himself every Friday night and which were followed by nearly debilitating flulike side effects that lasted through the weekends. "This medication changed my personality, making me irritable at best. Despite the routine, exacerbations continued, and my quality of life continued to deteriorate." One of Nick's later relapses affected the muscles of his eyes, leaving his vision blurred to the point that he "could no longer see to perform daily tasks."

Finally, Nick talked to his doctor about stem cell therapies, which he had seen described on the television news. After several referrals, in 2001, he ended up in Dr. Burt's office at Northwestern Memorial Hospital in Chicago. Unfortunately, at this time, Burt was performing bone marrow transplants only on severely handicapped MS patients, and so Nick didn't quite qualify. But Burt's trial passed the safety test with flying colors, and when the FDA deemed it ready for a more able-bodied population, Nick was first on the list for treatment.

"On July 1, 2003, I received my stem cell transplant," he wrote. "After four months devoted to my transplant and recovery, I went back to work symptom free in September of 2003." You'll recall that Nick had four flare-ups in five years, and that this number would likely have been much higher without escalating medications that altered his personality and lifestyle. As part of a five-year follow-up study, Nick reported being completely symptom free. "I look forward to continuing to live an active, productive, MS-free lifestyle that includes my work as well as playing racquetball, golf, and coaching hockey."

In a 2006 interview with the Health Radio Network, Nick simply said, "I'm very blessed. Very blessed."

It's tempting to call Richard Burt's treatment of Nick's multiple sclerosis a cure, but at a minimum it's a long remission.

Like the treatment for leukemia, destroying a patient's bone marrow (and thus his or her immune and blood system) and replacing it with a new one is an aggressive, risky therapy and is certainly not for every MS patient. In the period after the blood system has been killed and before the maturation of the new one, patients are desperately at risk for infection, and it's not unheard of for patients to die from the procedure before they would have been killed by multiple sclerosis.

So, in the mid-2000s, Burt refined his treatment so that he would not have to destroy a person's entire immune system. Instead of chemotherapy to kill the old system followed by a complete bone marrow transplant, maybe it was just that the immune systems of MS patients needed to be "reset."

Terrence McCann was one of the first patients to test the theory. In 2004, Terrence had been a star high-school football player when his season was cut short by what he thought was a bad sinus infection. He was tired, he was sick, and his vision was blurry. His cold cleared up, but the blurry vision remained. Eventually, Terrence was diagnosed with multiple sclerosis—his vision problems were caused by optic neuritis, the same inflammation of the optic nerve that Nick Blanchard had and that is common in MS patients.

Like most early-stage MS patients, the drug interferon controlled Terrence's symptoms for a while—in his case, two years—but then the disease started to overpower the drug, as it did with Nick and as it commonly does. Terrence needed a new drug. Only he was allergic to the next step up. What could he do? It looked like he was on an uphill treadmill, like Nick, of ever-stronger side effects for ever-stronger drugs that would, in any case, eventually be no match for the disease. Instead, he enrolled in the next generation of Richard Burt's MS clinical trial.

In this version, Burt and his team first used a drug to coax Terrence's mesenchymal stem cells out of his bone marrow and into his blood, where they then harvested these cells by drawing his blood and spinning it in a centrifuge to separate the stem cells. Then, instead of nuking Terrence's entire bone marrow blood system, they wiped out only the components of his *immune sys-*

tem before quickly reintroducing his own MSCs. Unlike a donor blood system that requires time to mature and take root, once thawed and injected, Terrence's own stem cells got right to work reconstituting his old immune system. But because these new immune cells were growing up from scratch (from stem cells), they didn't think that myelin was a foreign invader that needed to be attacked and destroyed. Instead, they recognized myelin as belonging to the same team they played for and left it alone. Scientists call this immune tolerance.

But the real question was whether the newly reset and "tolerant" immune system would pick up where the old one left off, chipping away at the myelin that insulated Terrence's axons.

Terrence told the *Saturday Evening Post* what happened: "I started to feel improvement while I was in the hospital. I realized that I didn't need my glasses to see. At home my parents noticed that my balance was improving and that I didn't seem as fatigued as before. Honestly, these changes started within the first month after coming home. My life continued to improve. By the third month, I was actually going to the YMCA to exercise."

In May 2009, the *New York Post* reported that Terrence McCann walked across the stage of Virginia Commonwealth University to receive an MBA in marketing. He had gone three years without medication and without symptoms. "It's a blessing," Terrence said.

Again, like Nick Blanchard, it's tempting to call Terrence's treatment a cure. (Doctors like Burt are too careful and/or too modest to use emotionally charged words like *cure*.) But Burt and colleagues reported their results in the January 2009 issue of the top-tier journal the *Lancet Neurology*, in which they wrote that after three years of follow-up checks, during a time in which you would expect the disease to progress and patients to become increasingly disabled, 17 of 21 patients who had treatment alongside Terrence in fact improved their scores on a standard disability scale. While patients should have been slipping downhill, they were instead climbing up. And of the four patients who didn't improve, none got worse. Not one patient in Burt's study showed disease progression, and 16 of the 21 patients were "relapse free," meaning that for at least three years, multiple sclerosis that tends to come and go in waves hadn't reared its ugly head.

Pardon the scientific jargon, but here is how Burt and his coauthors summed up their results in their *Lancet* paper: "Autologous ['from the patient'] nonmyeloabalative ['without killing the bone marrow'] haematopoietic stem cell ['blood-forming, adult stem cell'] transplantation for patients with relapsing-remitting MS with active inflammatory disease and frequent exacerbations is a feasible procedure that not only seems to prevent neurological progression, but also appears to reverse neurological disability."

In other words, adult stem cell treatment for early MS works and is far less risky than a full bone marrow transplant. And the number of patients with early MS undergoing this procedure is blooming exponentially. Richard Burt currently has the treatment in a phase III clinical trial, and all involved expect the treatment not only to gain FDA approval but to be covered by most medical insurances by the year 2015.

In fact, following Burt's 2009 *Lancet* article, a British team at the Health Economics and Decision Science Research Group of the University of Sheffield, United Kingdom, took up the question of the treatment's cost-effectiveness. Using a complicated mathematical model that compared cost to "patient-level data from registry sources," the study found that hematopoietic stem cell transplant "is estimated to cost below £3,000 [$4,700] per quality adjusted life year gained." They caution that without a large, randomized control trial, "conditions for comparative analysis were not ideal," and so this number is rough. Results were published in the June 2010 issue of the journal *Bone Marrow Transplantation.*

But despite the lag-time in FDA approval, the success stories of curing multiple sclerosis with immune system "reset" via mesenchymal stem cell transplants keep coming. In August 2011, 37-year-old MS patient Monterrey Potter from Melbourne, Australia, updated the results of her treatment with mesenchymal stem cells at the website http://www.msstemcell.com. A news video Monterrey posted to the site shows her in the hospital before her treatment, unable to walk and with a catheter to control her incontinence. Her young daughter says, "I missed Mommy!"

And the same video shows Monterrey months later, walking and riding an exercise bike. At her website, Monterrey lists the results of her treatment: "I no longer take any MS medication. MRIs have confirmed disease activity has stopped. My appetite is normal again. I am no longer wheelchair dependent and walk without aids. My incontinence has gone. My pain has gone. No more crying myself to sleep. I am driving again and my quality of life has improved beyond words. I am living life and enjoying being a mother to my child again."

In a world of maybes and almosts and in-the-futures, the treatment of early MS by harvesting and reinfusing adult mesenchymal stem cells is now an immediate, powerful treatment for many patients and a cure for some. The case of early MS is one in which stem cell therapy has proven its effectiveness and is elbowing its way into the mainstream.

"It's a miracle. It's incredible. It's surreal," Monterrey told the *Herald Sun.*

But you'll notice one little word in the preceding section that unfortunately makes a big difference, and that word is *early.*

Resetting the immune system with the transplant of autologous mesenchymal stem cells works spectacularly well to stop the immune system from doing more damage.

But multiple sclerosis is a disease with a tipping point. Nick Blanchard, Terrence McCann, Monterrey Potter, and the nearly one-thousand-and-counting patients treated with this stem cell method of resetting the immune system were in the "relapsing-remitting" stage of the disease. In this stage, the disability during flare-ups is followed by a remission. While damage may be continuing in the nervous system during remission, there is periodic return to normal or near-normal function. The trick is to stop the flare-ups and hopefully also stop the damage to the brain and spinal cord.

But there's another side of the disease, another stage called secondary-progressive multiple sclerosis, in which functions that are lost are gone for good. This transition from relapsing-remitting to secondary-progressive is a powerful tipping point. Every ratchet down the path of secondary-progressive MS is a ratchet that cannot be reversed. Or, at least not yet.

And now finally, we're back to Dr. Jeffrey Cohen at the Cleveland Clinic. In 2010, Cohen was enrolled in a phase I clinical trial that dips the first toe into the use of mesenchymal stem cell infusions in patients with secondary-progressive MS. And instead of blasting an immune system and then "resetting" it with stem cells to rescue the patient, Cohen is exploring whether stem cells can heal damage already done. "It's become evident that there is ongoing attempted repair via natural processes, but in most patients it's inadequate," says Cohen. "There's a great therapeutic need in MS to treat the degradation or to aid the repair, and that's where things like our approach comes in."

His first patient was forty-six-year-old Bob Harold of North Olmstead, Ohio, whose story was reported in the August 23,

2011, issue of the *Cleveland Plain Dealer*. Six years prior, Bob had been 233 pounds of muscle—the owner of a fitness gym and a flooring company—when he started noticing unusual fatigue and hugely uncharacteristic weakness. "My balance was off," he told the *Plain Dealer*. "[People] thought I was stoned at work all the time, or drunk. I don't smoke. I don't drink."

Eventually, in 2007 Bob was diagnosed with multiple sclerosis and started taking medications for the condition. But like so many people we've met in this chapter, the side effects were extreme. He dropped fifty pounds, and despite daily injections, the disease was winning the battle. Bob had tipped from relapsing-remitting MS into secondary-progressive MS. MRI scans revealed lesions in his brain—the scars created by the disease that are the most menacing sign of progression.

When Bob told Cohen he was done with drugs, Cohen brought up the subject of his new stem cell clinical trial. "I was just gung-ho on trying it. When you get this, you just want to be normal," Bob told the *Plain Dealer*.

First, Cohen and his team harvested a small number of mesenchymal stem cells from the bone marrow of Bob's hip. Then Cohen and his colleagues expanded these stem cells in the lab. (This sounds easy, but the ability to turn stem cells into more stem cells is actually not that easy. The Fred Hutchinson Cancer Research Center in Seattle published their technique in January 2011. Before this new technique, doctors could get stem cells to divide and mature in the process, but not multiply into many new stem cells. See chapter 14 on cancer for details.)

After three months of growing these stem cells, instead of killing Bob's immune system, Cohen and his team simply infused this now massive number of healthy mesenchymal stem cells back into Bob's blood through an IV in his arm. (Remember, they weren't trying to stop his immune system from eating away his nerves' myelin coating; they were trying to repair the damage his immune system had already done.)

A month after treatment, Bob told the *Plain Dealer*, "I used to have to use my left arm to lift my left leg up. Now I can lift [the leg] up on my own." Bob also reported increased stamina and improved eyesight. But most important, an MRI taken two months after the treatment showed that the progression of Bob's brain lesions had stopped.

Three other phase I trials in Spain and Iran are using adult mesenchymal stem cells to treat multiple sclerosis, and a fourth phase I trial, in China, is doing similar work with umbilical cord MSCs. "Not only can these cells improve repair in some tissues by turning into the cells of that tissue—bone, cartilage, skin—and not only do they also encourage existing stem cells by producing a variety of growth factors, but they also have useful anti-inflammatory properties," Cohen says.

Inflammation is the sign of the immune system attacking an invader—of B cells and T cells streaming to the site of an infection or, in the case of MS, gathering near a nerve fiber's myelin sheath for the immune system's mistaken cannibalization of needed tissue. "These mesenchymal stem cells appear to be able to migrate from blood into damaged tissue, where they modulate inflammation. They can seek out areas of inflammation or tissue damage and do their thing," Cohen says.

In fact, inflammation may play a role in Richard Burt's technique of immune system "reset." His theory is that a minitransplant of stem cells allows the "new" immune system to operate in an inflammation-free environment. That seems to let the newly reinfused stem cells to grow up realizing that the patient's myelin isn't a foreign invader, and so the autoimmune destruction of the nerve insulation stops.

Cohen calls this first clinical trial of stem cells infused through an IV for the treatment of secondary-progressive MS "pretty conservative" and hopes to use initial results like those of Bob Harold to expand into a larger trial. Still, Cohen says the treatment could be offered in a clinical setting within five to seven years.

Will a similar treatment save cosmetics mogul Victoria Jackson's daughter Emma? "Since my diagnosis freshman year, I've visited 34 doctors in over six different states. I've also had 58 blood draws, 17 MRIs, and 23 IV infusions," Emma wrote in a 2010 issue of her newsletter, the *SPECTRUM*, which is hosted at the website of the Guthy-Jackson Charitable Foundation (http://www.guthyjacksonfoundation.org). In that year, her senior year of high school, Emma got straight As, was the MVP of her extremely competitive tennis league in Los Angeles, and was the editor of her school newspaper.

On April 18, 2011, the University of Calgary in Canada posted the details of a new clinical trial of stem cell transplant for neuromyelitis optica—the same treatment that Richard Burt and others pioneered for multiple sclerosis.

On the Guthy-Jackson foundation's website in the spring of 2011, Emma wrote, "As I go off to college, explore new things, meet new people, and just enjoy being a kid, I know nothing can stop me—not even the fear of blindness or potential paralysis, because the cure will come." Then on September 17, 2011, vibrant, motivated, and intelligent Emma tweeted, "It's official, I've moved into college!! I can't believe it's finally happened!!"

With the world's best treatment, Emma's neuromyelitis optica remains in remission. With her mother's support, stem cell scientists are within a hair's breadth of a cure. While the scientific community is working hard to overtake MS through stem cell research and therapies, Emma and her relatives keep fighting, just like thousands of other people looking for the best clinical solutions.

Chapter 11

Arthritis

There are more than one hundred forms of arthritis, ranging from an octogenarian's creaky elbow to a life-threatening condition that attacks children before they even walk.

Let's start with a look at stem cell treatments for bread-and-butter arthritis—the kind that to some degree affects more than 70 percent of Americans older than sixty-five, osteoarthritis. The Center for Disease Control estimates that more than 22 percent of American adults have at least one arthritic joint—49.9 million people.

One of them is Sylvia Bell, who at age seventy-two was told she needed a double knee replacement to repair her severely arthritic knees. It's not an uncommon operation; in fact, in 2003 the National Institutes of Health estimated that 300,000 total knee replacement operations were performed, and in 2011, as the population aged and the technique improved, CNN estimated that more than 500,000 Americans had knee replacement surgery.

But what if you didn't have to lop off a major section of the longest bone in your body, or require a knee replacement surgery? In May 2011, ABC News reported that Sylvia decided to try an experimental stem cell therapy. At his clinic in Broomfield, Colorado, rehabilitation medicine specialist Dr. Christopher J. Centeno had performed the procedure on more than two hundred patients since 2009 as one of the several Regenexx stem cell programs he offers. In it, he harvests adult mesenchymal stem cells from a patient's hip, concentrates and expands these cells in the lab, and then injects them into the patient's arthritic joints. As opposed to three to five days in the hospital for a knee replacement, Centeno's stem cell treatment is an outpatient therapy, after which patients generally walk out of the clinic with a knee brace. ABC News reported that most patients were able to start rehabilitation within a week, which usually included stationary cycling. And as we know, autologous mesenchymal stem cell therapy—meaning cells from a patient's own bone marrow or blood—carries few risks. Unlike embryonic or induced pluripotent stem cells, when mesenchymal stem cells are infused into a patient, they're no more likely than the patient's existing cells to form tumors. ABC News quoted Dr. Centeno as saying, "Because the stem cells come from your own body, there's little chance of infection or rejection."

The results of Centeno's procedure are striking. He told ABC News that "two-thirds of [our patients] reported greater than 50 percent relief and about 40 percent reported more than 75 percent relief one to two years afterward." Two years after stem cell treatment, only 8 percent of Dr. Centeno's patients then decided to have knee replacement surgery. While not inexpensive, the treatment is less expensive than a knee replacement and rehabilitation. However, the technique requires expanding the number of cells, which necessitates costly clinical trials (as much as $50 to $100 million) before approval of the Regenexx technology. Because the procedure isn't FDA approved and insurance companies don't cover it, some patients choose "medical tourism," traveling to the Cayman Islands for treatment.

Still, patients like Sylvia Bell think it's worth the cost. When interviewed by ABC, Sylvia had just returned from a weeklong bicycling trip on which she had covered twenty to forty miles per day. And she did it without pain. "Almost from the moment I got up from the table, I was able to throw away my cane," she told ABC. "Now I'm biking and hiking like a thirty-year-old."

Rheumatoid arthritis, however, is a different beast entirely. Instead of the expected wear and tear of joints over time in os-teoarthritis, rheumatoid arthritis is an autoimmune condition in which a person's immune system attacks the joints. In many ways it's more appropriate to pair this with multiple sclerosis than with wear-and-tear arthritis. The language of rheumatoid arthritis is *synovial membranes*, *hyperplasia*, *ankylosis*, and *DAS28*. In contrast, the language of dancing is *arabesque*, *plié*, *sauté*, and *tours chaînés déboulés*. Elizabeth Embridge speaks both languages.

Now in her sixties, former dancer Elizabeth says of living with rheumatoid arthritis for forty years, "There are challenges every day—getting up, starting my day. I'm frustrated when I can't button certain things, when I can't zip things, when I can't dance like I used to be able to dance."

The National Institutes of Health estimates that 1.3 million people in the United States live with the crippling disease, and modern medicine does little more than hope to hold rheumatoid arthritis at bay. Treatments are like using a pole to hold back a fighting bull, which eventually, inevitably, snaps anything in its path on its way to your body. There is no cure.

Because rheumatoid arthritis is an autoimmune condition, to understand the disease you have to know a little bit about its instigator: the human immune system. Humans would be much better off if we could refrain from opening the hermetically sealed package of our skin—bugs would stay out, blood would stay in, and the nearly impervious barrier between the two would generally keep us free of disease. But humans don't stay in these healthy bubbles. Every day, in every corner of the world, we do unhealthy things like breathing and eating. We open our eyes to look around; we inject pathogens directly into our bloodstreams on the edges of imperfectly controlled steak knives; we fly in airplanes that recirculate air and hundreds of people's germs for hours; our kids sneeze in the backseat, and so while piloting an SUV on the interstate, we breathe in germs.

In short, every day we bombard ourselves with viruses, bacteria, and fungi. Luckily, the human immune system is built to fight off these assaults. When we ingest, insert, or inhale something foreign, our immune system recognizes, kills, and eliminates it. In fact, the immune system is made up of two parts—one unchanging immune system you're born with and an "adaptive" immune system that changes as you age to combat the bad guys that happen to invade your neighborhood.

Both immune systems depend on white blood cells, which come in many forms. For example, the innate immune system is made up of a number of different cells, which float around in the blood and tissues looking for foreign material. They have rather odd names like mast cells, phagocytes, macrophages, and granulocytes. When an infection occurs, these cells rush to the site, ganging up on any infectious material they find. This is why a cut gets puffy and why an infected cut leaks pus—these dead and dying white blood cells are the prime ingredient of pus.

The adaptive immune system is trickier. Yes, it remains dependent on white blood cells, but the adaptive immune system primarily uses a different kind of white blood cell known as a lymphocyte. Actually, there are two kinds of lymphocytes in the adaptive immune system: B cells and T cells.

B cells search for bad guys, and T cells search for cells that have been infected by bad guys, generally speaking. The result is the same: whether they're floating freely in your blood or whether they've already infected your body's cells, foreign bacteria, viruses, and other invaders are killed.

You don't want to be a foreign agent in your body. Equally bad is being perceived as a foreign agent. This is what happens in an autoimmune disease. For whatever reason, the immune system sees a patient's tissue as foreign and attacks it. While it's still unclear exactly why, in rheumatoid arthritis B cells and T cells attack joints. Actually, that's not quite true. Recent research shows that B cells and T cells don't actually do the attacking—it's not as if these cells are sharks clustered around the joint, eating away at it—but instead these lymphocytes are instrumental in misrecognizing joint tissue as foreign and then in helping create the body's erroneous immune response. B cells and T cells pull the handle that causes the cascade of inflammation that eventually degrades joints.

But while the exact science is unclear, the results of this misguided immune system are crystal clear: the synovial membrane that lines joints and the protective sheaths around tendons become inflamed, leading to all sorts of devastation in the affected joints. Patients lose cartilage. Bone erodes. And once something—whatever it is!—causes the immune system to attack this synovial membrane tissue, the immune system only learns to attack it more quickly and efficiently. Often it starts with the hands, progresses to the feet, ankles, and knees, and then starts to erode any and every synovial joint in the body. As an added bonus, chronic inflammation and the common therapies used to combat it can lead to lung fibrosis, kidney amyloidosis (protein deposits in the kidney), heart attack, and stroke.

Rheumatoid arthritis is a progressive, degenerative condition, and it is a condition with no known cure. A news release from the California Institute for Regenerative Medicine said, "When a combination of genetic propensity and injury to cartilage kicks off the changes that lead to arthritis, there is no way to halt it. Arthritis can also be triggered by joint infection, aging, or gout." Still, unlike many of the conditions described in this book, it doesn't necessarily kill, at least not quickly. Rheumatoid arthritis is a sentence for a long, painful life.

"Physically, I feel like it's a broken bone that never heals. It's just a constant ache," Elizabeth Embridge told HealthLine.

But rheumatoid arthritis isn't only a disease of the elderly. Mike Veldt of Spokane, Washington, was diagnosed with juvenile rheumatoid arthritis when he was nine months old. "There were times when he was younger when he couldn't walk and times when he couldn't crawl around," his dad told the *Spokesman-Review* in an article dated September 21, 2011. But this article is in the sports section. Rather than focusing on Mike's disease, the paper describes the boy as a six-five, 225-pound high school senior, fighting through the pain of what doctors at Seattle Children's Hospital described as "bone-on-bone contact" to star in football and wrestling at Mead High School. He is also a 4.0 student and scored 2130 out of a best possible score of 2400 on the Scholastic Aptitude Test (SAT).

In short, Mike is an outstanding young man with a very bright future ahead of him. Also ahead of him is the continuing, everyday fight of his life. He said to the *Spokesman-Review*, "I haven't let arthritis stop me, and I won't let it stop me. No excuses. It's not necessarily going to be easy at times, but I'll get through it."

It's only been two years, since his sophomore year, since he's had a major flare-up. He hopes to make it as long as possible without another. But they'll come. He knows it, and his doctors know it. And while juvenile rheumatoid arthritis (JRA) sometimes burns itself out in adulthood, it leaves crippled, devastated joints in its wake. The treatments for JRA can temporarily treat and/or mask symptoms, but they're no cure.

The California Institute for Regenerative Medicine offers another option. Its 2009 annual report, available online, describes it thus: "They're like biological M&M's—only very, very small ones—designed to treat arthritis. A shell of juvenile cartilage cells wrap a center formed of stem cells plucked from bone marrow."

This is a promising method of cartilage repair developed by Jeffrey Lotz, PhD, director of the Orthopaedic Bioengineering Laboratory at the University of California, San Francisco. Lotz wanted to use cartilage stem cells to repair tissue damage but couldn't find enough of them to do the trick. So instead, he went back a step to mesenchymal stem cells, the stem cells found in bone marrow (among other places). It's easy to harvest these cells but trickier to make them turn into cartilage instead of into fat, bone, or skin. "Thus the M&M idea arose," said the CIRM report. "The sheath of juvenile chondrocytes—cartilage cells—act [*sic*] like guides, sending signals that tell the stem cells, Hey, we're supposed to become cartilage."

Lotz mixes these cartilage-wrapped mesenchymal stem cells with biomaterial and then injects them into damaged tissue, where they work their magic, churning out cells to match their surroundings—in this case, their cartilage coats.

Or at least that's how it works in rabbits. The CIRM report said, "Whether they will work to replace native cartilage in weight-bearing joints awaits testing in larger animals."

In the meantime, for patients with advanced rheumatoid arthritis, there's the strategy that's been curing leukemia since 1968. Leukemia and rheumatoid arthritis are two very different diseases, but both result from white blood cells gone bad. In the case of leukemia, these white blood cells are cancerous, replicating themselves without restraint and eventually choking out the healthy white blood cells and other components of the blood system. In the case of rheumatoid arthritis, white blood cells have turned on a patient's body, eating away the synovial joints.

So it seems sort of logical that a treatment for leukemia might also cure rheumatoid arthritis.

We met Dr. Richard Burt, chief of immunotherapy for autoimmune diseases at Northwestern University, in our chapter on multiple sclerosis and other autoimmune diseases, and here is the reasoning he sets forth in a proposal (at ClinicalTrials.gov) for a clinical trial of bone marrow transplant for advanced, severe rheumatoid arthritis (so please pardon the science-ese):

> Rheumatoid arthritis (RA) is a chronic illness, immunologically mediated, probably induced by the exposure to an antigen or antigens, to which immunologic tolerance is lost. The disease has a variable course, from a mild, intermittently symptomatic illness requiring only symptomatic therapy to a fulminant illness requiring dangerous immunosuppressive therapy, surgery, or both. The molecular defect causing RA has not been characterized, but may involve aberrant T cell, B cell, and macrophage function. Although RA often responds to immunosuppressive medication including corticosteroids, methotrexate, azathioprine, and cyclophosphamide, or to nonsteroidal anti-inflammatory drugs, no therapy has been curative. In patients with severe RA, who have been unresponsive to

corticosteroids, and who have more than twenty active joints or vasculitis, we propose, as a phase I-II study, complete immune ablation and subsequent reconstitution with autologous in vitro T lymphocyte depleted PBSCs [peripheral blood stem cells] harvested from the patient prior to immune ablation. The combination of high dose cyclophosphamide and anti-thymocyte globulin conditioning will be followed by rescue with autologous lymphocyte depleted PBSCs.

Basically, Dr. Burt proposes an MS-like immune system reset, only this version is a full immune system wipeout and reconstitution, more like a stem cell transplant for leukemia—first knocking out a patient's malfunctioning immune system and then restarting it with stem cells harvested from the patient's bone marrow before the procedure.

In fact, Burt has worked with similar treatments since the early 2000s. In the August 2004 issue of the journal *Arthritis and Rheumatism*, Burt and his collaborators report the results of their stem cell transplant into a fifty-two-year-old woman who failed to respond to traditional rheumatoid arthritis treatments. At the time of her treatment, the woman had twenty-four swollen joints and thirty-eight "involved" joints. Instead of using her own stem cells, Burt harvested blood stem cells from her sister and then, after killing the patient's defective immune system, reconstituted it with stem cells from the sister.

Even before leaving the hospital, the patient's morning stiffness disappeared. At her nine-month follow-up visit, the fleshy tissue lumps of the woman's rheumatoid nodules were gone. A year after treatment, Burt wrote that "her RA has remained in remission with no immunosuppressive or immunomodulatory medications."

Much like T cells and B cells starting the cascade of the immune system's response, Burt's study initiated a cascade of similar studies, eventually published under such titles as "Sustained Remission, Possibly Cure, of Seronegative Arthritis after High-Dose Chemotherapy and Syngeneic Hematopoietic Stem Cell Transplantation" (McColl, Szer, and Wicks, *Arthritis and Rheumatism*, 2005). Or take a review published in the March 2011 issue of the journal *Current Stem Cell Research and Therapy*, whose authors wrote the following about young patients with juvenile rheumatoid arthritis who had failed other treatments: "For these severely ill patients autologous bone marrow transplantation (aBMT) is a last-resort treatment. [The] aBMT is remarkably effective in suppressing disease activity, with beneficial outcome reported in around 70 percent of these previously refractory patients. Moreover aBMT is the only treatment that can induce a lasting medication-free disease remission in these patients."

A press release from the Arthritis Foundation, summing up what these findings mean for patients, quoted Dr. Daniel Lovell, a pediatric rheumatologist at Cincinnati Children's Hospital Medical Center, saying, "I would say that with the information we have at this time, stem-cell transplantation may have been a cure for some of the patients." However, the risk involved with killing the immune system—leaving patients temporarily exposed to any and every infection—means that the procedure itself can kill. The Arthritis Foundation release said that "because of these risks, death occurs in 5 to 15 percent of all stem-cell transplants."

This aggressive reset of the immune system is not for everyone. Of the people who undergo the treatment, somewhere in the neighborhood of 1 in 20 will die of complications. But for rheumatoid arthritis patients who have reached the end of the line of traditional therapies, whose bodies are otherwise strong enough to withstand the assault of chemotherapy and radiation treatments, this replacement of their malfunctioning immune system with their own adult, mesenchymal stem cells is tantalizingly close to a cure.

Chapter 12

Scleroderma, Lupus, and Other Autoimmune Conditions

In the past few chapters, we've seen stem cells treat and even cure diseases like multiple sclerosis and rheumatoid arthritis. Here we'll see that these are not the only autoimmune disease patients who can benefit from stem cell therapies—either stem cell infusions that act as booster packs or the immune system reset of chemotherapy followed by stem cell transplant.

"Seven years ago, I had a comfortable, happy life. I was working part-time as a nurse, pregnant with my second child, and living in the suburbs with my husband. I was looking forward to a long, wonderful future," Debbie Marks wrote on the website of Northwestern University's Feinberg School of Medicine. Then, "six years ago, I was diagnosed with scleroderma."

Scleroderma literally means "hard skin." It is an autoimmune connective tissue disease affecting blood vessels and collagen production, in which the body's immune system attacks and kills supple tissue and replaces it with ropes of collagen. It is more common in women than in men. In the skin, it's the difference between silk and twine, and in the case of scleroderma, as skin tissue becomes hard collagen, it hardens and tightens.

Eventually, living in your own skin becomes like wearing shoes three sizes too small. Maybe an ancient echo of this experience or something similar is described in the passage of Job 19:20, which states, "My bone cleaveth to my skin and to my flesh." The systemic form of the disease also affects internal organs like the heart, gastrointestinal organs, and even kidneys and lungs.

Debbie wrote:

As the disease progresses, your organs can grow hard and thick. The skin on your face gets so taut that it can drastically affect your appearance. You can lose the ability to chew and to close your mouth. It can change the way you speak. The skin on your hands can get so tight that your fingers become fixed in a clawed position, completely useless. You can lose the ability to walk. The blood vessels can narrow, resulting in a loss of circulation [a condition known as Raynaud's disease]. Raynaud's can lead to painful sores that can take years to heal and often result in amputations. The digestive tract can become inflamed, causing heartburn and eventually the inability to eat. The GI tract can become affected, leading to malabsorption of nutrients, diarrhea, and constipation. Your kidneys can fail. Muscles and joints can become inflamed and painful. The lungs become stiff, making it difficult and eventually impossible to breathe. Your heart can become scarred and weak, making it unable to efficiently pump.

The Scleroderma Foundation estimates that three hundred thousand people in the United States live with scleroderma and that a third of these people have the systemic form of the disease. It tends to run in families, though no genes controlling the disease have been discovered, and for unknown reasons it tends to attack women more often than men (though affected men have worse prognoses). The disease includes forms that span the spectrum of severity, running from a localized skin condition that tends to clear up on its own to the progressive, systemic form for which the five-year survival rate is only 50 percent.

Unfortunately, that latter, aggressive form of the disease is the one that attacked Debbie Marks. According to the Mayo Clinic's website, "scleroderma has no known cure—no drug will stop the overproduction of collagen."

And so Debbie's disease progressed. "Five years ago I was 'living' with scleroderma," she wrote.

My face was so tight that I couldn't bend my head backwards. It was getting hard to keep my mouth closed. The ligaments in my gums were weakening, causing all my teeth to loosen....I could not raise my arms above my head. When I tried, it felt like the skin on my abdomen was ripping. I could not make a fist, cross my fingers, or whistle. I could no longer button or zipper, tie shoes, do my girl's hair, floss my teeth, cut up food, or open any jar. My fingers were so sensitive that turning on a light was painful. Not an hour went by that I wasn't somehow reminded of my disease and my limitations.

And then a year later, skin became the least of Debbie's worries. Scleroderma attacked her lungs, replacing the expanding and contracting endothelial cells with unforgiving collagen and reducing her lung capacity by 67 percent. As surely as if she'd looked at Medusa, Debbie was turning to stone.

"I wrote a letter to my husband to let him know that it was okay to love again, that it was okay to let the girls call another woman 'Mommy,'" she wrote. "Afraid I would never see the Magic Kingdom [through] my children's eyes, we took a trip to Walt Disney World. I was running out of hope for the future. I was slowly dying."

Debbie enrolled in a clinical trial with Dr. Richard Burt at Northwestern University. We've seen Burt's immune system "reset" elsewhere, and this was the treatment if not of choice then of last resort for Debbie. On March 2, 2007, Burt and his team injected Debbie with drugs that encouraged her bone marrow to release mesenchymal stem cells into her bloodstream. These stem cells were then harvested by hooking her up to something called an apheresis machine. (Not as scary as it sounds—it's like the machine that's used when you donate platelets. It takes blood from an IV in one arm, spins out the stem cells, and returns the rest of the blood through an IV in the other arm.) Then Burt and his team killed Debbie's existing immune system with chemotherapy and radiation and then reinfused the stem cells, which went to work creating the components of a new blood and immune system—an immune system that would tolerate Debbie's own tissues (see page 119) and not mistakenly attack them.

"It was twenty-nine days of rigorous but hardly insurmountable treatment," Debbie wrote of her experience on Northwestern's website.

Before her treatment, Debbie's lung function had been spiraling like a penny in a funnel down toward that black pinpoint of nothing. Six months after her treatment, not only had the spiraling stopped, but her lung function had improved from 43 to 57 percent.

"I could make a fist again," she wrote. "I could lift my arms up high and drop my head back without a problem. I could button my own buttons and help my kids get dressed. I could fix their hair. I could help them bathe. I could go up a flight of stairs. I could chase my kids around the park. I went back [to] work."

And in 2011, four years after treatment, Debbie's lung X-rays read as normal. "Today, I have hope that I will see my daughters' recitals, proms, and weddings.... I have hope that I will celebrate my fiftieth wedding anniversary.... Today, because of my stem cell transplant, I have a comfortable, happy life. Today, I am looking forward to a long, wonderful future," she eloquently wrote.

As of the fall of 2011, the only other place in the country running clinical trials of autologous bone marrow transplant for scleroderma was the Fred Hutchinson Cancer Research Center in Seattle. In the 1970s, "the Hutch," as it's known, pioneered the use of bone marrow transplants for blood cancer patients and, along with Northwestern, has been pushing the treatment into autoimmune diseases.

One of the Hutch's first patients was Susan Branford, a data-billing clerk from Inchelium, Washington, a small town on the Colville Indian Reservation. According to a 2003 article published in the Fred Hutchinson magazine *Quest*, Susan's symptoms started with tingling in her toes but quickly progressed through extreme hot/cold sensitivity to systemic scleroderma that attacked her lungs. Without a cure, doctors prescribed increasingly strong regimens of anti-inflammatories, which they hoped would suppress or at least dull her body's mistaken immune response. When her disease continued to progress, Susan ended up at the Hutch.

"None of the medications I had tried was working," she told *Quest*. "The treatment at Fred Hutchinson was my last chance."

In this early iteration of the treatment, after killing Susan's immune system with chemotherapy and radiation, Dr. Richard Nash jump-started her system with stem cells donated by her brother—the traditional "matched donor" approach that doctors at the Hutch had long used for leukemia. Six months later, Susan's lungs had begun to heal. The 2003 *Quest* article stated that "more than three years post-treatment, the scleroderma—hardening of the skin—has almost gone away, except for the skin on her fingers. And she has regained enough energy to return to work."

Again, the treatment is not for everyone. For example, if scleroderma has given you a mild skin rash, there's no need to obliterate your immune system over it. Likewise, if your disease is responding to traditional drugs and therapies, the risk of infection inherent in the stage between the death of the old, faulty immune system and birth of the new one makes this stem cell reset more dangerous than it's worth.

"These are considered pilot studies and are for patients who have failed other therapies and otherwise probably would have a 50 percent risk of mortality or severe disability," Dr. Nash told *Quest.*

Back to Northwestern, where Katie Haskell describes her experience with another autoimmune disease, lupus. Like scleroderma, lupus can affect only the skin or can be systemic throughout the body. Like rheumatoid arthritis, lupus leads to chronic inflammation that attacks any and every body tissue, in this case including the brain. Current treatments can help slow the pace of the disease, but there is no cure.

In 1978, Katie was nineteen years old and working a college summer job as a waitress, when her hands inexplicably swelled. She went to the University of Michigan Hospital emergency room in Ann Arbor and was soon diagnosed with lupus.

Though anti-inflammatory drugs kept the disease partially in check, over the next twenty years her immune system slowly ravaged her body. "I have had two mini strokes, which affected my speech and right side of my body. Twenty years of steroids left me at 254 lbs., severely [Cushingoid], with cataracts, and osteoporosis. I had vasculitis on the brain and central nervous system involvement," she wrote.

When she finally made her way to Dr. Richard Burt's clinic at Northwestern, the disease had eroded her once whip-smart brain, leaving her with a functioning IQ of 80, which is in the realm of mild developmental disability. "Many times when I left the house I could not find my way home or remember where I lived," Katie wrote.

And like Debbie Marks's scleroderma, Katie's lupus had eroded her lungs, leaving her with 18 percent of normal lung function and dependent on an oxygen canister twenty-four hours a day. Most people with this lupus-generated form of pneumonia die within ninety days. "I was dying," wrote Katie. "My doctor, one of the top ten lupus doctors in the world, had run out of ideas."

It was then, in 1998, that Katie became one of the first patients to undergo immune system reset at Dr. Burt's clinic at Northwestern. Her treatment was nearly identical to Debbie Marks's, and her results followed a similar trajectory as well.

By 2008, when Katie wrote the retrospective of her disease to post to Northwestern's website, her lupus was exactly that: a retrospective. In 2006, she earned an associate's degree in science with honors and then transferred to the University of Michigan bachelor's degree program in nursing. The university's graduation records show that Katie earned her nursing degree with honors in 2009.

Dr. Burt and his colleagues followed seven similar lupus patients for up to three years after autologous stem cell transplant. One way to measure lupus is by the diversity of patients' T cells. This is because as the disease progresses, T cells tend to not only attack patients' tissues but become increasingly *specialized* to mistakenly attack these tissues—instead of a mix that keeps patients safe from many diseases, T cells become a homogeneous bunch that can attack only the patient. After chemotherapy and rescue with autologous stem cells, the level of T cell diversity in these seven patients returned to healthy levels. In fact, not only did all seven patients stabilize their conditions and not only did they improve their T cell diversity, but all seven continuously improved to the point of remaining free from active lupus even without accompanying treatment with immunosuppressive medications.

Of course, a promising study leads to more studies, and after seeing the results of Burt's seven-person lupus treatment, the FDA authorized a larger trial. This time Dr. Burt and his Northwestern colleagues treated fifty patients, and the results of their five-year follow-up were published in the February 2006 issue of the highly respected *Journal of the American Medical Association* (*JAMA*). As with the first study, the patients in this expanded trial were those with systemic lupus that hadn't responded or had stopped responding to all other treatments. In this group, stem cell therapy was a treatment of last hope, without which almost all would certainly soon have died (untreatable lupus in the 1950s was a death sentence for almost all patients within five years). Yet in their *JAMA* article, Burt and collaborators reported that at the five-year point, 84 percent of these patients were still alive. Not only that, but a full 50 percent of them, who were supposedly beyond hope, achieved "disease-free survival."

Again, doctors tend to err on the side of caution and would rather not call this a cure. But to anyone without an MD or an MD/PhD behind their name, "disease-free survival" sure looks like one.

Through the late 2000s, researchers at Northwestern, Fred Hutchinson Cancer Research Center, and elsewhere have continued to refine this likely cure. For example, giving drugs to an autoimmune disease patient that encourage their bone marrow to release mesenchymal stem cells into the bloodstream where they can be easily harvested sometimes has the unexpected consequence of creating disease flare-ups. And also, when you harvest this stem-cell-rich peripheral blood, even after purification, in addition to the stem cells you want, samples tend to include remnants of the original immune system's T and B cells that were creating the problem in the first place. Or in addition to bad cells being reinfused into a patient, the DNA of a patient's stem cells may predispose them to redevelop the disease. And a final major problem with this technique is the difficulty in getting enough stem-cell-rich blood to quickly rescue patients whose immune systems have been killed.

For all these reasons, it would be great to be able to grow transplantable stem cells in the lab. You wouldn't have to use drugs that risk generating flare-ups; you wouldn't give back remnants of patients' original, faulty immune systems; and you could theoretically grow as many blood stem cells as you want, allowing doctors to infuse their patients with a quantity of blood that would allow the immune system to reboot quickly, rather than leaving them at terrible risk of infection for a month or more.

So, the pie in the sky for current researchers is discovering how to move these autoimmune treatments from autologous (again, from the patient's own body) to allogeneic (transported from elsewhere). One way to do this is by using the bone marrow stem cells of a matched donor—but there remains the chance that a patient's body will reject this donated blood. Worse yet, the new immune system could actually try to reject its new host, a potentially lethal complication called graft-versus-host disease (GVHD).

So, as another option, the National Institutes of Health describes researchers' attempts to grow blood stem cells in the lab. An article on the NIH's website (http://stemcells.nih.gov) said, "In the future, scientists may be able to modify human stem cell lines in the laboratory by using gene therapy or other techniques to overcome this immune rejection. Scientists might also be able to replace damaged genes or add new genes to stem cells in order to give them characteristics that can ultimately treat diseases." Some researchers are looking to use T cells rather than stem cells to reset a person's immune system, such as Jeff Bluestone, PhD, who is working on diabetes at the University of California, San Francisco.

Another autoimmune disease firmly in the sights of stem cell therapies is type 1 diabetes. In the case of type 1 diabetes, the immune system mistakes the body's insulin-producing beta cells of the pancreas as foreign and attacks them. In the healthy body, when these cells detect sugar, they release insulin, which tells the body's cells to take up the excess sugar and store it, thus keeping blood glucose levels within pretty narrow limits. In type 1 diabetes, without the ability to make insulin, blood glucose levels roller-coaster between two very unhealthy extremes.

This may be a bit harder to picture than being squeezed to death by one's own skin (scleroderma) or detaching control signals from muscles (multiple sclerosis) or the immune system eating joints (rheumatoid arthritis) or the immune system eating everything (lupus), but the result is the same: without treatment, patients with type 1 diabetes die, but first they suffer kidney failure, painful feet, amputations, strokes, heart attacks, and blindness.

Fortunately for these patients, treatment has been around for some time in the form of purified pig insulin and, more recently, genetically engineered synthetic human insulin shots. If your immune system has killed your pancreas's ability to make insulin, you can inject insulin as needed. But this requires constant vigilance and turns patients into human pincushions. If just once a patient with type 1 diabetes forgets to inject insulin, blood glucose can spike, leading the body to try to cleanse this glucose through urine and scrubbing the body clean of much of the water and salts it needs to function. Even worse in the short term is injecting too much insulin, which can lead to dangerous hypoglycemia, low blood sugar that can cause coma and even death.

Also, without insulin, the body switches to exclusively burning fatty acids—a strategy that evolved to add a little more energy in times of low blood sugar levels rather than to provide the body's sole source of sustenance. Exclusively burning these fatty acids quickly leads to the accumulation of their waste product, acidic ketone bodies, which lower the blood pH level. This is why diabetics in crisis start to pant—hyperventilation helps the body offload carbon dioxide and blood acidity along with it. But finally, with continued lack of insulin, the body's compensatory machinery is overrun, and diabetics can lapse into coma, which before insulin treatment was almost always fatal.

Even without the extreme case of life-threatening diabetic coma, if patients fail to precisely control their blood glucose levels over time, complications are likely, including kidney failure, heart disease, blindness, stroke, nerve pain, and amputations.

If you are diabetic, don't cheat on your diet and don't skip your injections.

Recently, researchers have worked with pancreas transplants or replacing the pancreas's insulin-producing beta cells. But according to the World Health Organization, there are between 11 and 22 million people living with type 1 diabetes worldwide, and there aren't nearly enough donated pancreases to go around.

So in the spring of 2007, when Northwestern's Richard Burt reported success in "curing" diabetes with the immune reset we've seen elsewhere in this chapter, the results were reported by all the major news sources, including "Diabetics Cured in Stem-Cell Treatment Advance" (the *Sunday Times*), "Adult Blood Could Yield Stem Cells to Treat Diabetes" (CNN), "Stem Cell Experiment Lets Diabetics Forgo Insulin" (MSNBC), "Study: Stem Cells May Reverse Type 1 Diabetes" (*Time*), "Stem Cells—A Possible Cure for Diabetes" (ABC), and "Stem Cells Offer Hope for Diabetics" (CBS).

As you could probably tell from the headlines, autologous stem cell transplant after immune system suppression does good things for patients with type 1 diabetes. Burt's was a study of fourteen young people with early-onset type 1 diabetes and was conducted in Brazil in collaboration with Dr. Julio C. Voltarelli of the School of Medicine of Ribeirão Preto at the University of São Paulo. At the time of treatment, all of the fourteen young patients required daily insulin shots. After treatment, one went a month without insulin, another went five months, seven went at least six months, four went at least twenty-one months, and one patient went thirty-five months without needing an insulin shot.

In a 2009 interview with *Time* magazine, Burt said, "It appears we changed the natural history of the disease. It's the first therapy for patients that leaves them treatment-free—no insulin, no immune suppression for almost five years."

In 2009, researchers discovered a new type of stem cell in amniotic fluid—one harvested by trapping excess fluid after birth. These AS cells can birth insulin-producing pancreatic beta cells. When these lab-grown beta cells are immersed in glucose, they produce insulin, and when glucose is scarce, they stop. There are a number of steps between the lab and the clinic, and students have begun by injecting these stem-cell-engineered beta cells into pancreases of diabetic mice.

Still another approach looks at type 1 diabetes not as a problem of an overall faulty immune system but of an immune system out of balance. You see, there are actually two kinds of T cells: ones that attack invaders and ones that regulate these attackers. These regulatory T cells, or T-reg cells, tone down their aggressive T cell brothers and sisters. And so biotechnology companies like Athelos, a subsidiary of NeoStem, are exploring type 1 diabetes and other autoimmune diseases as conditions of imbalance. By harvesting and expanding T-reg cells and then infusing this riot police back into patients' overeager immune systems, they can quiet down the overactive immune response and restore balance to the patients' systems. In fact, the technique of harvesting, expanding, and reinfusing T-reg cells is set to start clinical trials soon.

More recently, researchers have recognized a new way to address type 1 diabetes. Recall that in type 1 diabetes, the body's own immune system turns on itself and wipes out the insulin-producing beta cells in the pancreas. As we discussed, this may be the result of an imbalance between our T-reg cells and aggressive T-effector cells. While this imbalance exists, it has hampered the ability of researchers to successfully transplant new beta cells from humans, which are in limited supply in the pancreas.

A new approach is being developed by Islet Biosciences. The company recognized early on that human type 1 diabetics use bovine (cow) insulin as a replacement and inject it often multiple times daily. (Today, most diabetics use genetically engineered human insulin.) As it turns out, pig (porcine) insulin is nearly identical to human insulin, too. Islet Biosciences is developing porcine beta cells encapsulated in alginate (a porous protective bubble), where they can live, read the sugar levels in the surrounding environment, and produce insulin as needed. The insulin itself is small enough to travel through the pores of the bubble and into the body. The destructive antibodies, however, cannot pass through the bubble and as such do not destroy these cells.

Animal studies with this technology have shown promising results, and the company is planning to initiate the first human trials in 2013.

So, the story of autoimmune diseases is one of a stem-cell Baskin-Robbins with far more than thirty-three flavors. Some treatments are but a twinkle in an innovative researcher's eye, others are springing from the lab into mice, and still others are working their way through human clinical trials. And some have made the transition from science fiction to nonfiction. An August 2011 review published in a respected German medical journal (in reference to a study originally published the year before in the journal *Haematologica*) writes the following summary:

> Over 1,500 patients worldwide have received a hematopoietic stem cell transplant (HSCT) as treatment for a severe autoimmune disease. Most of these have been autologous and mostly have occurred in the past 15 years . . . A recent retrospective analysis of 900 patients showed that the majority had multiple sclerosis (n=345) followed by systemic sclerosis [scleroderma] (n = 175), systemic lupus erythematosus (n = 85), rheumatoid arthritis (n = 89), juvenile idiopathic arthritis (n = 65) and idiopathic cytopenic purpura (n = 37). An overall 85 percent 5-year-survival and 43 percent progression-free survival was seen, with 100-day-

transplant-related-mortality (TRM) ranging between 1 percent (rheumatoid arthritis) and 11 percent (systemic lupus erythematosus and juvenile idiopathic arthritis). Around 30 percent of patients in all disease subgroups had a complete response, often durable despite full immune reconstitution. In many, e.g., systemic sclerosis, morphological improvement such as reduction of skin collagen and normalisation of microvasculature was documented, beyond any predicted known effects of intense immunosuppression alone.

This review article confirms that treating people with severe autoimmune diseases with their own hematopoietic adult stem cells is a valid therapy.

The treatment of autoimmune diseases, mostly by autologous stem cell transplant after immune suppression, is not pleasant. But it works. And the continuing work of Richard Burt at Northwestern, Richard Nash at Fred Hutchinson Cancer Research Center, researchers at Wake Forest, the NeoStem subsidiary Athelos, and the many, many other doctors and scientists who punch a clock in labs around the country and around the world will ensure that the plusses continue to go up while the minuses continue to go down, extending the umbrella of stem cell treatment over more and more patients whose risk/reward scales currently leave them in the cold rain of disease progression.

On July 29, 2010, Debbie Marks, the first patient we met in this chapter, wrote, "It has been more than three years and I am doing great. My lung studies continue to be stable and the inflammation in my lungs remains gone. I am back to work and I am still trying to catch up with my girls. I am back to living my life and appreciating all of it. (OK, sometimes—after a particularly long day with a certain 10 year old and 6 year old clawing each other's eyes out—I have to remind myself to appreciate ALL of it.) I am 100 percent sure that the stem cell transplant saved my life!"

In a photo that accompanies the post, Debbie smiles at the camera with her family, hugging kids on either side of her, her husband looking like he just ran into the frame after pushing the camera's auto-shot timer. Her younger daughter has a hula hoop hanging over her shoulders. Her older daughter looks like, *OMG! I totally can't believe you made me stand in this picture, Mom!* And Debbie looks beautiful and strong in sandals and a beaded necklace, reading glasses pushed up on her short black hair.

After writing a letter to her husband and girls with instructions and advice for after she was gone, now, down to the last imperfect detail, everything in Debbie Marks's life is back to being exactly as it should be.

Chapter 13

Cosmetics

Who doesn't want to look younger? Americans spend nearly $2 billion on antiaging creams and another billion on Botox treatments geared toward removing wrinkles and defying gravity. A recent online shopping search shows an ounce of name brand "un-wrinkle" cream selling for $150. Among other active ingredients, the cream contains a chemical that the product maker claims "mimics the venom of the Temple Viper, which has been proven to be very effective in blocking muscle contraction."

Literally, this is snake oil.

And if you think the traditional cosmetics market is full of fast pitches for miracle antiaging creams, try Google-searching *stem cells cosmetics.*

In fact, by law none of these cosmetic products are allowed to contain human cells of any kind, including stem cells. If any such claims were true, these products wouldn't be cosmetics; they would be drugs, and that would mean roughly $100 million in testing needed to push through the FDA approval process.

More logical than these creams but equally unproven through traditional and clinical trials are face-lifts that harvest stem cells from fat in the body and inject them through the epidermis into

various regions of the face, most using a procedure very similar to injections of Botox. But like anything else in medicine,
before making claims of proven benefits, trials need to be completed and the results published in peer-reviewed journals.

The premise makes sense. For years, cosmetic surgeons have
been transplanting fat from one part of the body to another, but
without adequate blood supply the transplanted tissue dies. If
transplanted with stem cells means new blood vessels form to
nourish the fat with oxygen and nutrients, reason stands that this
could work. Physicians who feel they should be allowed to treat
patients under the practice for medicine believe a therapy will
work.

The "why not try it?" approach of the few face-lift clinics
promoting the procedure disregards the risks. According to an
article in the journal *Nature*, "Of the roughly 60 peer-reviewed
articles on mesotherapy [cosmetic injections into subcutaneous
fat] published within the past two decades, more than half focus
on complications and unwanted side effects, including delirium
with psychotic features, facial cutaneous ulcers, and multifocal
scalp abscess with subcutaneous fat necrosis. No study has
yet focused on stem-cell-based mesotherapy, although doctors
in Thailand are sounding the alarm about a potentially deadly
treatment offered there that allegedly removes facial wrinkles
with injected animal stem cells. Several doses, a doctor told
Bangkok's *Nation*, could lead to fatal anaphylactic shock."

Simply: yikes.

Still, the promise of stem cells for cosmetic treatments is al-
luring. Could stem cells be used to grow new, youthful skin?
Yes, definitely—see this book's chapter on burns. Could stem
cells someday be used to plump up lips or breasts without
surgery? Almost certainly. In an interview with ABC News, Dr.
Peter Costantino, formerly director of the Center for Facial Re-

construction and Restoration at Roosevelt Hospital in New York and now director of the New York Head & Neck Institute, sums up the current state of things, saying, "You can't just inject 'fat' stem cells into a breast and just assume that it's going to make a nice-looking breast. You could just end up with something fairly lumpy and unappealing."

Jeremy Mao, director of the Tissue Engineering and Regenerative Medicine Laboratory at Columbia University's College of Dental Medicine, is pioneering stem cell technology as a complement to reconstructive surgery. In fact, in addition to the use of stem cells to create completely new skin for burn patients or in cases of scarring, the area of cosmetics that has made the most use of stem cell technologies is dental medicine. In a 2008 review for the *New York State Dental Journal*, Mao writes, "MSC-derived chondrocytes can be used for reconstruction of orofacial cartilage structures, such as nasal cartilage and the temporomandibular joint. MSC-derived osteoblasts (bone-making cells) can be used to regenerate oral and craniofacial bones. MSC-derived myocytes (muscle cells) can be used to treat muscular dystrophy and facial muscle atrophy. Stem cell-derived adipocytes (fat cells) can be used to generate soft tissue grafts for facial soft tissue reconstruction and augmentation." While these terms are a little specialized, the point is this: adult mesenchymal stem cells can regrow almost all the components of the human face and dental systems.

And now we're firmly back to the realm of scientific tissue regeneration instead of pseudoscientific cell plumping and wrinkle smoothing. Most of the techniques Mao describes are pushing their way toward clinics, but let's take a closer look at just one of these uses of stem cells with reconstructive surgery.

When you lose a tooth to decay, disease, or trauma, the bone that once supported it starts to shrink. Left long enough, the bone shrinks to the point that implanting a new tooth becomes impossible. To counteract this, surgeons can sometimes perform an operation called a sinus lift in which bone is grafted into the area of the molars and premolars. Then again, sometimes they can't.

Dr. Russell Taichman at the University of Michigan, in partnership with the biotechnology company NeoStem and with funding support from the US Department of Defense, is exploring the use of VSELs in increasing the speed and success of bone healing. Another biotechnology company is working with the University of Michigan researchers to see if bone marrow stem cells will increase the speed at which healing occurs in sinus-lift operations. Basically, the hope is that these cells, in conjunction with a cocktail of growth factors, will grow new bone in the graft site, providing the bedrock needed for dental implants.

Areas that toe the line between traditional cosmetics and medicine have hope for stem cell cures. Take the research of Iran's Royan Institute with autologous ("from the patient") transplantation of stem cells into vitiligo patients. Vitiligo is the unsightly loss of pigment cells in the deep layers of the skin, leaving irregular, milky white patches of skin surrounded by normally pigmented skin. It's especially disfiguring in African-American skin, in which the contrast between light and dark is particularly stark. It's the condition that led Michael Jackson to use bleaching agents on his dark skin to try to match the white areas that had lost their pigment.

Published in a 2010 issue of the journal *Archives of Dermatological Research,* the Iranian team showed that of ten adult patients with stable vitiligo, six months after treatment, four had a marked response (76 to 100 percent reduction in vitiligo patches), two had a moderate response (51 to 75 percent), two had a mild response (26 to 50 percent), and two showed minimal response, with 20 percent reduction in the size of their vitiligo patches.

This is a treatment of the present, with the authors writing, "This method is an effective, simple, and safe therapeutic option for stable vitiligo lesions." For between $2,000 and $3,000, vitiligo patients can have this procedure done at the Royan Institute in Tehran or at a handful of clinics around the world. A clinical trial of the procedure in the United States has been approved by the FDA. The Henry Ford Medical Center in Detroit conducted a similar, FDA-approved clinical trial, with results expected soon.

But as for the traditional definition of cosmetics, as in creams that turn back the clock on aging, you'll have to wait.

Chapter 14

Cancer

In 1845, pathologists Rudolph Virchow and John Hughes Bennett fused the Greek words *leukos* (meaning "white") and *aima* (meaning "blood") to describe the blood of a cadaver who, when examined, looked as if its veins flowed thick with pus. (Like many cancers, the realities of leukemia make for poor dinner conversation.) There are many kinds of leukemia, but all are blood cancers, pure and simple—the result of a single cell in which random genetic mutations allow it to produce offspring that replicate out of control.

There are a number of "leukemia movies." Some, like *My Sister's Keeper*, raise important moral dilemmas. Some show a great concern about environmental pollution and its impact on health, like *A Civil Action*. Others emphasize love and the power of changing people, like *A Walk to Remember*. But in all of them there is an open drama of sickness—a clear picture of leukemia.

What is leukemia about? It is a story about blood, where whichever type of blood cell that has become cancerous squeezes other, healthy cells out of existence. Patients with reduced platelets bleed uncontrollably. Patients without white blood cells are prone to infections and sores. Patients whose red blood cells have been squeezed from the system become ane-mic. Whatever the specifics, leukemia cells soon become the blood system's dominant life-form, and without treatment, it is universally fatal.

Approximately every four minutes, one person in the United States is diagnosed with a blood cancer, and every ten minutes, someone in the US dies from a blood cancer. This statistic represents nearly 145 people each day, or more than six people every hour. The Leukemia and Lymphoma Society estimates that within the United States alone there are almost 275,000 people with leukemia, and more than 44,000 new cases were diagnosed in 2011. These numbers should make us think, also because according to the American Cancer Society, new global cancer cases could increase to 21.4 million by 2030.

Cases of leukemia are particularly difficult, partly because you can't surgically remove the affected tissue as you can with other forms of cancer. Instead of living in a defined, operable tumor, the cancerous cells flow throughout the body with your blood—and surgeons can't hit moving targets. So the only treatment for leukemia is to target the cancerous cells with chemotherapy and radiation, to scorch the field that is a patient's blood system in hopes of killing leukemia before it kills the patient.

But, for many reasons, blood is obviously a good thing to have inside your body. And so after killing a leukemia patient's blood system, doctors have to build a new one. Though they didn't know it at the time, in 1968 when doctors at the University of Minnesota performed the first successful bone marrow transplant on a child suffering from a disease of the immune system, they were using stem cell therapy.

At the core of your bones is the marrow, and this marrow produces the components of your blood system, including the red blood cells that carry oxygen and the white blood cells that keep your body clear of disease and infection. The factories within bone marrow that do the actual work of creating blood are stem cells. And in a patient whose blood system has been obliterated by chemotherapy and radiation, it's a transplant of these bone marrow stem cells that can regenerate a new blood system. With precision, skill, and more than a touch of luck, since 1968, doctors around the world have refined this technique of bone marrow transplantion to point the way to health for between 20 and 75 percent of patients diagnosed with leukemia (prognosis depends on a range of risk factors).

On the morning of August 13, 2011, at the University of Colorado Hospital outside Denver, Amy Thoreau got a different kind of bone marrow transplant. Twelve weeks prior, she had visited her doctor feeling fatigued, weak, and without appetite. At the time, Amy was twenty-four weeks pregnant with her sixth child and worried her symptoms were the result of complications. Unfortunately, it wasn't her child making her unusually lethargic; it was leukemia, and she needed treatment right away. But the toxic radiation and chemotherapy cocktail would kill her baby. Amy was faced with an excruciating dilemma: "Do I care more about this unborn baby? Do I care more about myself? Who do I save?"

Amy decided to save her baby. She delayed her own treatment in order to carry her child to viability. Her son, Ronin, was born tiny but healthy at twenty-nine weeks. Only then, desperately behind the survival curve, did Amy check herself into the hospital for the start of a last-ditch treatment to save her own life.

At the CU Hospital, medical oncologist Dr. Jonathan Gutman immediately set about the hard work of annihilating Amy's leukemia, bombarding her with chemotherapy and radiation, killing the cancer cells but at the expense of her immune system.

Ten weeks into the treatment, Amy was left with almost nothing—few red blood cells, white blood cells, or platelets, and almost no healthy bone marrow to make more . . . but also without leukemia. Her blood system had been nearly erased, deleted from her body.

And now is when Amy and Dr. Gutman stepped off the path of traditional treatment. You see, there remain problems with the way bone marrow transplant is usually done. First, you need to find a donor who matches a patient's ten critical tissue markers—too little match results in graft-versus-host disease, in which the new blood system battles the patient's body, and it can be like trading one vicious, degenerative, and frequently fatal disease for another. Seventy percent of Caucasian patients but only 10 percent of African-Americans can find an adult blood donor in existing banks.

On the flip side, a donor's blood needs a small degree of *mismatch* with the patient's blood so that the immune system of the new blood recognizes any lingering bits of the old blood as different from itself and so wipes out all remaining traces of leukemia. Otherwise, if the new blood is too perfectly matched, residues of leukemia can remain and lead to relapse.

Of course, you can hope to avoid relapse by completely obliterating the original blood system, but the more aggressive this chemotherapy and radiation, the higher the chance this toxic treatment will kill a patient as horribly as does the disease. Finally, and important, in the window between the death of the old, leukemic blood system and the birth of the new one, patients without immune systems are at terrible risk of infection and disease. Until a patient's bone marrow stem cells start spitting out the leukocytes and lymphocytes that are the body's white blood cell assassins, patients are solely dependent on antibiotics, antivirals, a perfectly sterile room, and commonly a pain pump to ease the excruciating experience of living somewhere between living and dead. In this window, a visitor's sneeze can be lethal.

And so the common bone marrow transplant for leukemia is a life-and-death balancing act of complications in which doctors try to match a patient's condition, progression, genetics, and demographics to the treatment that does the most good while doing the least harm. In other words, after a diagnosis of leukemia there is no good scenario, only a scenario that chooses the best of the bad.

In 1988, researchers took another step toward the goal of a treatment for leukemia without life-threatening side effects when doctors in Paris, France, infused a six-year-old child suffering from an autoimmune disease with stem cells from umbilical cord blood. Cord blood transplants have one major advantage over blood transplants from an adult donor: they needn't match nearly as well.

"The baby's blood system has to coexist with the mother's in utero," says Jonathan Gutman, Amy Thoreau's doctor and investigator at the University of Colorado Cancer Center, "and so this cord blood has evolved to remain compatible with many blood systems." Instead of needing to match ten critical tissue markers, cord blood may need only to partially match six markers in order to avoid the complication of graft-versus-host disease.

But like blood from a perfectly matched donor, because this blood acts so benignly once transplanted, it frequently fails to compete with and thus eradicate the remaining traces of leukemia from the original blood system. So, the common practice is to infuse patients with *two* units of umbilical cord blood, each from a different cord. The blood from these separate cords competes with the remnants of the original blood, and that's when things turn ugly. "What we postulate is that there's a battle between the two cord bloods, making one more able to knock out not only the other cord blood, but also the remaining leukemia," Gutman says.

It's a bit like making someone want to date you by introducing them to a potential rival.

But here's the major problem with cord blood transplants, even *double* cord blood transplants: you just don't get enough blood cells. An umbilical cord is not a large thing, and it doesn't contain much blood. And so in the period while the cord bloods are battling for dominance and then repopulating the immune system cells needed to fight fungus, virus, and bacteria, the patient is desperately fragile—horribly susceptible to every infection that blows through the room.

"It takes a long time for stem cells to start growing again," Gutman says of traditional double cord blood transplants, "and patients sometimes go forty-five days without an immune system. It's miserable, and during that time patients are vulnerable to infection. That prolonged period has contributed to the largest problem with cord blood transplants: early transplant mortality, dying from complications."

According to Dr. Gutman, the bottom line on bone marrow transplant from an adult donor versus double cord blood transplant is that "there's an increasing body of evidence that they do equally well, but the way you get to survival is different. Cord blood offers a lower level of relapse, but higher mortality after transplant."

The answer seems easy: just use the original cord blood and grow it in the lab until you get a number of stem cells comparable to what you'd get with an adult donor.

Only it's not that easy. The catch is this: while you can grow cord blood in the lab, it increases the number of blood cells but not the number of stem cells. "Sure, you can grow a stem cell into six million neutrophils [one of the white blood cells that target bacteria], but then twenty-four hours after I stick them into you, they're all dead," Gutman says, and there are not enough factories cranking out replacements.

You can grow blood, but you can't grow blood stem cells.

Again, until now.

Cells learn things by waving around proteins on their outer membranes, like sea anemones searching the ocean for bits of edibles. By waving these tentacles, cells learn what's floating around, allowing them to act according to their environment. One of these anemonelike proteins is called notch, and when a certain notch grabs a certain floating goodie, it makes stem cells create more stem cells. Gutman knows this because he did a postdoc fellowship at the Fred Hutchinson Cancer Research Center in Seattle, where researchers discovered the procedure.

"Now when we expand cord blood, we take out the cord blood stem cells and grow them in the presence of this ligand [goodie]," Gutman says. "Before this technique, researchers considered a tenfold expansion of stem cells highly successful, and now we're getting a hundreds-fold expansion."

Thanks to this development, Amy Thoreau didn't have to choose between the possible relapse of matched adult blood and the wretched infections that can follow a double cord blood transplant. Now, with this new technique of expanding cord blood stem cells, the double cord blood kills the remnants of leukemia while the teeming mass of its lab-grown stem cells quickly repopulates the immune system.

Amy could have spent forty-five days with no immune system, hooked to a pain pump and always a bacterium, virus, or fungus away from the end of her life. But because Jonathan Gutman knew how to grow cord blood stem cells in the lab, she walked out of the hospital eleven days after her transfusion. She went back to her family without leukemia and with the very real expectation to continue her life where it left off with her diagnosis twelve weeks before: as a vibrant mother of five, now six. Rather than the black bat of leukemia circling her head, her worries could go back to the baby's sleep schedule, her kids' school and sports activities, and whether or not she could find babysitters.

Because of stem cells and the University of Colorado Cancer Center's Jonathan Gutman, for Amy Thoreau, it was back to normal. She was the eleventh person in the world to receive this treatment, and while it's still early, the technique seems to be working well with all eleven.

Amy's is a great story, but her leukemia is only the first tale in what could be an entire book of stem cell treatments for cancer. Instead of diving into a catalog of the many ways in which stem cells can regrow systems and tissues killed by cancer and its treatments, let's look for a minute at the dark side of stem cells. Let's go to what may be the root of all cancer: just as stem cells can grow healthy tissues, so too can mutated stem cells grow tumors.

Early detection, prevention, surgery, chemotherapy, and radiation: these have been the focus of the National Cancer Institute since its founding in 1937. The NCI's 2010 budget was $5.1 billion, and over its seventy-plus-year history the treatments borne of the NCI have made certain cancers curable. For example, the diagnoses of Hodgkin's disease; prostate, testicular, and breast cancer; and many leukemias are no longer immediate death sentences. However, once cancer reaches a critical tipping point, all the brainpower, all the dollars, and all the technology of the NCI may be able to extend a patient's life only by months you can count on your fingers and toes. Despite seventy years and uncountable dollars, cancer still has no cure.

Targeting cancer stem cells may be that cure.

These cells may make up only 1 to 3 percent of a tumor's weight, a tiny fraction of the tumor itself, but whereas regular cancer cells may divide a few times and then die, these cancer stem cells churn out cancerous progeny indefinitely. When researchers inject regular cancer cells into mice whose immune systems are designed to allow cancer growth, these cells soon sputter, flicker, and die out. But introduce cancer *stem cells* in these same mice, and you soon have tumors . . . and dead mice. Likewise, with radiation, chemotherapy, and surgery, you may kill 99 percent of a tumor, but if you fail to kill the tumor stem cells, these cells can and do quickly repopulate the tumor. Many researchers believe these cancer stem cells are the root of the disease and especially the root of most relapses.

Dr. Max Wicha, director of the University of Michigan Comprehensive Cancer Center, says, "The identification of cancer stem cells means we have to fundamentally change the way we approach cancer treatment. Up to now, cancer treatments have been designed to shrink cancers down. And what we're finding is these traditional cancer treatments are able to kill the bulk of the cells in the cancer, but that the cancer stem cells are resistant to common treatments like chemotherapy and radiation therapy. If we're going to cure the more common cancers, we're going to have to find a way to eliminate the cancer stem cells."

Rather than indiscriminately carpet-bombing the body with toxic therapies, the new wave of cancer treatments is to identify and selectively kill the cells that give rise to cancer. And this is true across all types of cancer. "What we learn about one kind of cancer stem cell applies to other cancers," says Wicha.

Finally, after developing treatment after treatment that tries to cut a head off the hydra that is the many types of cancer, we may finally have dug down deep enough to take the monster at its body or heart. Cancer stem cells may be at the root of all cancers.

Unfortunately, these cancer stem cells are especially hard to kill. In fact, they are so resistant to chemotherapy and radiation that the doses needed to kill them leave behind only the husk of the patient. In other words, most bodies can't tolerate the chemotherapy needed to kill cancer stem cells.

Researchers at UCLA's Eli and Edythe Broad Center of Regeneration Medicine and Stem Cell Research studied what makes brain cancer stem cells so immortal, much like the proverbial cockroaches that, along with Tupperware and Twinkies, common opinion holds would be the only things left after nuclear war. One thing these brain cancer stem cells do very well is switch their energy source. They can go from burning glucose to "oxidative phosphorylation," which uses oxygen to help them survive toxic conditions.

"We found these cancer stem cells are substantially different in their metabolic states than the differentiated cancer cells they create, and since they act differently, they can't be killed in the same way," says Dr. Frank Pajonk, an associate professor of radiation oncology at UCLA and senior author of the study describing this finding, which was published in the September 2011 issue of the journal *Proceedings of the National Academy of Sciences*.

The point is that these cancer stem cells are distinctly tougher than regular cancer cells. But the difference that makes them tough may also be their Achilles' heel. As the saying goes, any nail that sticks up will be pounded down, and by noticing what makes cancer stem cells different from their neighbors, researchers may be able to target these differences to pound them down.

One person doing just this is Antonio Jimeno, MD, PhD,

and one of Jonathan Gutman's colleagues at the University of Colorado Cancer Center (also one of the country's most exciting cancer scientists younger than forty). Jimeno recently opened a clinical trial at the CU Cancer Center with the very realistic goal of knocking down the bulk of a tumor with the traditional chemotherapy drug cetuximab (brand name: Erbitux), while killing cancer stem cells with a hedgehog.

A hedgehog? In January 2009, other researchers wrote about this hedgehog in the journal *Nature*. Basically, in every stem cell in our body, there is a hedgehog that tells it what to do. In fact, this bossy cousin of the Southeast Asian moonrat isn't specific to humans—from fruit flies to Albert Einstein, the Hh signaling pathway (nicknamed "hedgehog") first tells the body how to develop. The Hh signaling pathway tells an embryo which cells should expand out into neural tissue or bones or organs.

Because the hedgehog signaling pathway tells stem cells what to become, a faulty hedgehog can tell stem cells to become cancerous. The biotechnology giant Curis and its partner, Genentech, are targeting faulty hedgehogs for destruction (note to those concerned for animal safety: please remember these are not *actual* hedgehogs). Specifically, the Genentech hedgehog inhibitor called vismodegib passed a 104-person safety trial and was approved by the FDA for the treatment in adults of basal cell carcinoma, a form of skin cancer.

Other targeted cancer stem cell therapies are even closer to the clinic.

Do you remember how Jonathan Gutman grew healthy stem cells in the presence of a "notch ligand" to tell umbilical cord stem cells to grow more stem cells for transplant into leukemia patients? Well, just like hedgehog, notch is another signaling pathway—one that tells stem cells to produce more stem cells. When scientists at Fred Hutchinson Cancer Research Center discovered this, they learned to make more stem cells. And knowing notch may allow researchers on the flip side to *keep* stem cells from growing. Take away the notch, and you take away stem cells' ability to reproduce themselves. At least that's the goal of the partnership between biotechnology company OncoMed and pharmaceuticals juggernaut GlaxoSmithKline. The dynamic duo has two notch-nixers in clinical trial and many more in the pipeline.

If it turns out that cancer stem cells have beards and healthy cells don't, we can learn to yank on these beards. If cancer stem cells have trick knees, researchers can kick them. In fact, the idea of Achilles' heels that are unique to cancer stem cells and so making them susceptible to targeted therapies is a massive paradigm shift in the way we think about cancer. Now, instead of blasting the body with toxic chemotherapies, the wave of the future is to send in the small, nimble strike forces of targeted therapies to selectively weed out cancer cells. And this targeted, individualized approach is even being tried in leukemia, the great stronghold of scorched-earth medicine.

In October 2008, Maria McKinsey of Orange, California, was looking over a cliff into a terrifying chasm. For five years she had been fighting the disease polycythemia vera, which starts with the explosion in production of red blood cells but then 15 percent of the time switches to the overproduction of white blood cells, which looks almost exactly like leukemia. In the fall of 2008, Maria's body was producing 95,000 white cells per cubic millimeter of blood, far above the normal 8,000 or so.

"I was headed down the leukemic path," she told the California Institute for Regenerative Medicine. Blood tests confirmed it: the sleeping lion of Maria's disease had woken up on the wrong side of the bed, and what was once polycythemia vera now looked like cancer. She was forced to use a walker, and her knee was making bone marrow outside the bone tissue—ramping up to create even more white blood cells.

And unfortunately for Maria, doctors couldn't find a matched bone marrow donor. Leukemia without a transplant is almost universally fatal. End of story.

That is, until Catriona Jamieson, MD, PhD, director of the stem cell research program at the Moores Cancer Center at the University of California, San Diego, tacked on another chapter. In 97 percent of patients with Maria's disease, the stem cells that cause the explosion of red and then white blood cells share the same genetic mutation—the same something that makes them different from all the other healthy cells in the body. In the case of polycythemia vera, this mutation is in something called the JAK-2 gene. And so as a last hope for Maria and fifty-nine other patients, Jamieson used a drug that turned this gene off. Without their teeth—this one mutated gene—the stem cells that had been haywire had no bite.

"Within two months I went from using a walker to a cane to walking on my own," Maria told the California Institute for Regenerative Medicine (CIRM). Her white blood cell count dropped to normal. After forty years, she rekindled a relationship with a high school sweetheart.

Maria's response wasn't a fluke. Another patient, a tall, handsome man named Saban, took the podium to speak with CIRM doctors about his polycythemia vera, explaining, "I went on the trial because otherwise it was an end-game scenario." Like Maria McKinsey, Saban had very quick results. "I was the second person to use this product, after mice," he says, "and my spleen started getting smaller; I could roll over and sleep on it." Standing at the podium next to Saban, Dr. Jamieson pointed out that Saban had tools in the front pocket of his jeans, and Saban said yes, in the last couple months he'd gone back to his hobbies of boatbuilding and sailing.

Another patient, Carl, told the CIRM doctors that after Dr. Jamieson initially told him he could not be accepted for the clinical trial, "Being a man of faith and a born-again Christian, it's kind of difficult to go to my maker and say, I need to be sicker, Lord." The clock ticked, the clinical trial wore on, and Carl got sicker. Finally, on the last day of the trial, Jamieson called Carl for one last shot to see if he qualified. With the trial closing in a matter of hours, doctors rushed Carl's bone marrow biopsy to the lab, where they found that finally he was, in fact, sick enough for the trial. "That was a Thursday, and on Monday I started taking the drug," Carl said. "Before the trial, my wife said my spleen looked like a football. I thought it looked like a big mackerel, you know, for deep-sea fishing, something big, meaty. Well, that's what was lying on my stomach. Wednesday I looked at my spleen, and it was smaller. Seven days after starting the drug, my spleen had gone away—went from 21 centimeters to 10. My liver had gone from 10 to 3 in a week. And I'm very, very grateful for that change."

Of the fifty-nine patients in this study, which was only supposed to show that the drug was safe, all stopped making abnormal white blood cells. All of their spleens shrank by half or more, back toward normal size. In half of the patients, spleen size returned to normal.

"It's exciting and kind of unexpected," Dr. Jamieson told CIRM. "This was supposed to be a safety trial. I thought it would be too little too late. I didn't think the results would be so good."

So we've seen bone marrow stem cells used to regrow immune systems killed by chemotherapy, we've seen cancer stem cells as targets, and we've seen gene therapy in stem cells that tweak the proteins they produce. Now get ready for one of the most fascinating uses of stem cells you'll see in this book.

In 2010, doctors in Seattle gave Ellie Kranzyk two months to live. "It's a short time when they tell you that, wow. You wouldn't even believe how short it feels," Ellie told CBS News. Forty-four-year-old Ellie, a substance abuse counselor, volunteered for the Seattle group Seal Sitters, watching beaches around Puget Sound to ensure that beachgoers don't disturb newborn seal pups. In March 2009, she had been diagnosed with glioblastoma, an aggressive and incurable type of brain cancer that even with the best care carries with it only a 26.4 percent two-year survival rate. Now, a year later, doctors told Ellie there was nothing they could do.

This is partly because brain cancers are especially tricky—many of the best chemotherapeutic drugs can't cross the blood-brain barrier, and even if they *could* cross, the brain frequently can't withstand the collateral damage caused by these powerful drugs. In the brain, tissue that is killed stays dead, and so some of the best, most toxic cancer therapies can't be used.

And so being confronted with an absolute worst-case scenario, Ellie decided to become patient number one in a revolutionary clinical trial. Here's how it worked:

Stem cells are the body's engine of repair, and so somehow they've evolved ways to know where repair is needed. Though researchers don't understand exactly how, wherever there's damage, that's where the stem cells go. This includes tumors. So doctors at City of Hope Hospital in Duarte, California, injected Ellie's brain with 10 million of her own neural stem cells, which migrated to the tumor site and attached themselves to cancerous cells.

Here's where it starts to get special.

Before injecting these neural stem cells, doctors had genetically engineered them to carry a special package—the ability to make a benign little protein. Then the patient takes a pill, which is also a benign little chemical that easily crosses the blood-brain barrier. But now, crossing independently, the neural stem cells and the pill have smuggled into the brain two pieces of a powerful weapon. When the pill hits the protein made by the neural stem cells, the two combine to form a powerful poison—and because the neural stem cells have hooked onto tumor cells, this poison most powerfully kills only these cancer cells.

For Ellie Kranzyk, it was too late. She died on Christmas Eve, 2010. Friends at Seal Sitters, where Ellie volunteered, wrote, "One of our most vivid memories of Ellie is one evening on Alki Beach: Ellie, all smiles, was wrapped up in a blanket on a camp chair, washed in the pink afterglow of the sunset—prepared to stay for hours if necessary, looking after seal pup Spike who was still on the beach (thankfully, Spike returned to the Sound around 9 p.m.). We were so privileged to share the beach with Ellie."

But Ellie had taken this first step on the moon. After her pioneering treatment, the therapy went into a clinical trial with sixteen patients newly diagnosed with glioblastoma. The results were nothing short of miraculous. Historically, 61.1 percent of these patients should have lived for one year—with this trial's combination treatment, 100 percent survived the year. Historically, only 26.5 percent should have made it two years—at two years, 80 percent of these patients were still alive. The treatment *tripled* the time of progression-free survival. At the time of writing, three of these sixteen patients, previously given only months to live, were free of the disease. It's too soon to tell whether this treatment is a cure or a temporary fix, but all sixteen of these early patients were given years of life, and three of the sixteen may now have to start worrying about things like cholesterol and achy joints—the trappings of old age they never thought they would see.

On January 19, 2011, the biotechnology companies NeoStem and ImmunoCellular teamed up to launch a phase II study of this therapy in nine clinics around the country (number NCT01280552 at ClinicalTrials.gov). The companies hope to expand this trial to twenty or more clinics and to treat two hundred patients. In preparation, they have selected a commercial manufacturer (Progenitor Cell Therapy) for large-scale quality processing to ensure that even though a person's own cells are used, they become part of a therapy that will be safe and have a consistent effect from person to person. Ellie Kranzyk's courage will almost certainly save two hundred years of life and could save many, many more.

Because of the cancer stem cell therapies in this chapter, patients like Saban have gone back to building and sailing boats. Carl no longer sleeps with a mackerel on his stomach. Maria put her walker in the attic. And Amy Thoreau can be a mother to her six children.

In cancer, these new therapies save lives.

"This is a godsend; that's all I can say for it," says Maria McKinsey.

Chapter 15

Sickle Cell Anemia

Has there ever been a more accurately named disease than sickle cell anemia? In it, crescent moons bounce through a patient's bloodstream, hooking on to each other like the tails of plastic monkey-in-a-barrel toys. These chains form nets, and the nets block blood vessels, leading to intense pain, stroke, heart attack, and tissue death, often including kidney failure. The average life expectancy for a woman with the disease is forty-eight and for a man is forty-two.

These sickles come from genetically defective stem cells in a patient's bone marrow, which produce the scythe-like red blood cells. The genetic defect is most common in people of African and Mediterranean descent, and the National Institutes of Health estimates that 1 in every 500 African-American children will be born with sickle cell anemia, making more than 80,000 cases in the United States and millions of cases worldwide.

Basically, patients with sickle cell anemia need healthy red blood cells. Traditionally, the way to get these cells is through transfusion—when normal red cell counts get low, patients get a boost in the form of donated blood, sometimes as frequently as every six weeks.

Another way to get this healthy blood is to trick the body into restarting production of fetal hemoglobin. Late during their time in the womb, all babies make this protein, which very effectively grabs oxygen from Mom's blood and transports it around baby's body. Since 1995, patients with sickle cell anemia have taken the drug hydroxyurea to trick the body into making this fetal hemoglobin, which picks up some of the oxygen left behind by their own sickle-cell red blood.

Sickle cell patients also tend to take copious amounts of antibiotics to help faltering immune systems deal with infection. Prophylactic doses of penicillin have reduced childhood deaths from infections like pneumonia. Still, especially in Africa where the disease may be underdiagnosed and undertreated, many children whose deaths are attributed to malaria or dysentery or pneumonia are in fact casualties of sickle cell anemia.

This imperfect landscape was the backdrop for grandmother Paula Crane's 2011 speech to an audience of doctors and researchers from the California Institute for Regenerative Medicine.

"I'm going to tell you a little bit about my grandson Andrew," Paula said. "He's really doing . . . okay." When Andrew was born, he was immediately tested for and diagnosed with sickle cell anemia. Because babies' blood is still rich with fetal hemoglobin, there's commonly a window after birth with no complications that lasts until fetal hemoglobin gives way to the sickle cells of a baby's own blood system. When Andrew's fetal hemoglobin gave out, his sickle cells quickly hooked on to each other like a tangle of fishing tackle, blocking a blood vessel in his brain. At nine months old, Andrew had a stroke.

"Normally when babies cry, their arms are moving, their legs are moving," says Andrew's grandmother. "I saw him the next day, and his right side was silent."

The day after his stroke, Andrew started the common, aggressive treatment for sickle cell anemia, including penicillin, hydroxyurea, drugs for iron overload, and transfusions as needed to give him enough normal blood cells to compensate for his defective ones. Now in elementary school, the treatment holds Andrew's sickle cell anemia at bay. "He wears a brace on his leg, he rides his two-wheeler, he handles the medication well, and [he] understands why he has to take the medication and why he has to go to the doctor every six weeks for a blood transfusion," his grandmother told CIRM.

Until recently, this limbo of symptom management has been the best option for patients like Andrew. And this is despite the fact that bone marrow stem cell transplant cures sickle cell anemia. More than two hundred children have been cured of sickle cell anemia by wiping out their blood system with chemotherapy and radiation and then restarting the system with the bone marrow stem cells of a matched donor. New stem cells mean new red blood cells.

But, especially for the African-American population that is so affected by sickle cell disease, it can be horribly difficult to find a matched donor. There are more than 9.5 million people in the Be The Match bone marrow registry, but only 7 percent are African-American. This means that while Caucasians have a 93 percent chance of finding a matched bone marrow donor, African-Americans have only a 66 percent chance of finding a match.

There is no match for Andrew.

But even with a match, bone marrow transplant is reserved only for the most robust patients with the most extreme cases of sickle cell anemia. As you probably guessed, this is a nasty catch-22—very rarely are sickle cell patients also robust enough to withstand the obliteration of their blood system and replacement with a new one. As we've seen elsewhere in treatments for leukemia, lupus, rheumatoid arthritis, and other blood diseases, this treatment is brutal. In the window between blood systems, patients die—especially if they have any additional organ dysfunction, as is almost always the case with sickle cell anemia patients. This is why of the more than two hundred cases in which bone marrow transplant *has* been used to cure sickle cell anemia, all have been children—only in young children has aggressive sickle cell disease not had enough time to decay organs past the point they could withstand a transplant.

So with a lack of matched donors and side effects that can be deadly for already sick patients, most sickle cell anemia patients struggle through life with Andrew's combination of medications and transfusions.

Not Amanda Morehouse.

Despite suffering from sickle cell anemia since childhood, in the early 1990s the tall, beautiful Amanda was a model, posing for covers and photo spreads in dozens of magazines. In 1996 she graduated from Livingstone College in North Carolina with degrees in sociology and business. Then, by the time she was forty, Amanda was on dialysis, the result of red blood cells blocking blood vessels in her kidneys and eventually destroying them.

In a 2010 article, the *Salisbury Post* reported that during a visit to the National Heart, Lung, and Blood Institute in Bethesda, Maryland, for a study on pulmonary hypertension, Amanda joked with her doctors about her failing body, saying that maybe she needed a stem cell transplant. Again, by the time a sickle cell anemia patient reaches twenty, let alone forty, their organs—like Amanda's—have usually sustained enough chronic damage that they are unlikely to survive a bone marrow transplant. Amanda's joke was little more than offhand wishful thinking.

But the National Institutes of Health was exploring a new approach, and when Amanda joked about her need, doctors at the hospital took her seriously. She became one of the first ten patients to undergo a new stem cell therapy for sickle cell anemia. Instead of killing her entire blood system, NIH doctors used light chemotherapy to tone it down a bit. Then they infused Amanda with fifteen thousand blood stem cells collected from her sister, Nieda, whose relevant genes were a 50 percent match to Amanda's.

Interviewed by the *Salisbury Post* in the weeks just after her treatment, Amanda said, "I have to have faith. That's what all the prayers are for—a cure."

Her prayers were answered; fifteen thousand stem cells is an infinitesimally small number when it comes to a transplant. But healthy red blood cells last longer than sickle cells—an average of 120 days, compared to only twenty or so days for a defective cell. And so even a small population of healthy stem cells allows the body to slowly but surely replace sickle cells with healthy ones, because these healthy cells outcompete their underperforming rivals. Six months after her mini transplant, Amanda's new stem cells were making 72 percent of her red blood cells. Two years after treatment, in nine out of the ten patients the transplant blood had taken over red blood cell production completely—there was no trace of sickle cells or their defective stem cell parents. Stem cell therapy completely cured Amanda and eight others of sickle cell anemia.

In December 2009, the NIH published the results of this ten-person trial in the prestigious *New England Journal of Medicine*. If you or a loved one suffers from adult sickle cell anemia, you can find the continuing version of this study at http://www.clinicaltrials.gov by searching for the study number NCT00977691.

Researchers at the California Institute of Regenerative Medicine are taking another step toward the ease of stem cell treatment for people like Andrew and Amanda. By snipping bad genes and inserting good ones into sickle cell patients' bone marrow stem cells, CIRM doctors hope that someday soon they will be able to harvest, fix, and reinfuse just enough of a patient's own stem cells to allow these reengineered cells to outcompete their defective neighbors. As Amanda showed, only fifteen thousand fixed stem cells might be enough. And if doctors could reengineer a patient's own stem cells, there would be no chance of rejection and no need for a chemotherapy knock-down of any sort. The treatment could be used even with the most fragile sickle cell patients—of which there are many.

The past was awful, the present is manageable, and because of stem cell therapies, the future is bright for patients with sickle cell anemia. Speaking about Amanda's trial, the National Institutes of Health researcher in charge of the study, Dr. John Tisdale, said, "Our patients have had a remarkable change in their lives. They are no longer being admitted to the hospital for frequent pain crises; they have been able to stop chronic pain medications, go back to school and work, get married, and have children."

After her treatment, Amanda Morehouse is back to her life. Soon, a stem cell treatment could give Andrew a life he's never had.

Chapter 16

Sensory Impairments

On May 8, 1922, the French Impressionist painter Claude Monet wrote to his friend that because of the encroaching blindness from cataracts, "I was forced to recognize that I was spoiling [my paintings], that I was no longer capable of doing anything good. So I destroyed several of my panels. Now I'm almost blind and I'm having to abandon work altogether. It's hard but that's the way it is: a sad end despite my good health!" Eyedrops prescribed by the French ophthalmologist Charles Coutela had brought only temporary relief. And Monet knew the story of fellow painter Mary Cassatt's disastrous cataract surgery in 1913 that left her effectively blind.

In fact, cataract surgery dates back to the Indian surgeon Sushruta, who, in the sixth century BCE, used a curved needle to push patients' clouded lenses around to the back of their eyes and out of their fields of vision. In 1748, French surgeon Jacques Daviel was the first to pull cataracts out of patients' eyes.

In 1923, Monet had little choice but to follow Daviel's lead, finally allowing his ophthalmologist to remove the cataract-choked lens from his right eye. Despite writing to his doctor, Charles Coutela, in the painful days following the surgery, "it makes me sorry that I ever decided to go ahead with that fatal operation—excuse me for being so frank and allow me to say that I think it's criminal to have placed me in such a predicament," Monet healed, regaining the sight in his right eye almost completely.

That's how eye surgery should work: people have problems, they have surgery, and they're cured—even if they remain a bit cranky about it.

In 2002, artist Virginia Doyle was diagnosed with an even more debilitating disease. Virginia's work had been shown in galleries from Paris to London to New York, and now macular degeneration was extinguishing the light of her world as surely as if it were pushing the slider down on a dimming light switch.

"I don't try to do what I can't do, but what I can do, which is to use colors I enjoy in new ways," she told the *Bookshare Blog*. "Sometimes, in rare moments, I lose track of my everyday world and slide into a euphoria of my inner self filled with imagination and a love of life. Now that macular degeneration has progressed to a stage where I am legally blind, I see less of my work and rely on the way it feels."

Macular degeneration comes in two forms—wet and dry—and is the leading cause of blindness in people older than fifty in developed countries. Like cataracts, macular degeneration results in a growing cloud over the field of vision, but macular degeneration works in a very different way. Normally, every day, you lose the top cells of your retina, the light-sensitive part at the back of your eye. The cells die, and their husks are eaten by the cells that live directly underneath them. Tomorrow's cells form at the same rate that today's die, so over time you end up with exactly the same, ever-renewing eyeball.

That is, unless like Virginia Doyle and two million other Americans, you have macular degeneration, in which the second layer of cells lose their hunger. In macular degeneration, these second-layer cells don't eat yesterday's dead husks, and so these husks accumulate. In addition to the cell shells themselves (which are even more difficult to pronounce if you're selling them at the seashore), these dead cells hold accumulations of the day's junk—the toxins and irritants that these cells can't help but pick up. And so not only do the husks block incoming light, but the accumulation of their toxins starts to eat away at the healthy tissue that surrounds them.

Eventually these toxins make eyes bleed. This is when dry macular degeneration becomes the wet form of the disease. The transition is a mixed curse and blessing—in wet macular degeneration, leaky blood vessels quickly destroy sight, but this wet form of the disease is treatable.

In dry macular degeneration, antioxidants like lutein and zeaxanthin have been shown to slow the disease a bit, doing a little of the eye's toxic waste cleanup. And ten years ago, transplanted cell layers taken from the eyes of cadavers looked like a possible cure, that is, until almost all transplants were rejected by patients' immune systems (there's no bank of matched-donor eye cells like there is with bone marrow). Recently surgeons tried another approach: harvesting healthy second-layer cells from elsewhere in the eye and transplanting them underneath the decaying tissue. But there just aren't enough cells in the eye to make this practical. Another approach has been to surgically lift the retina off the degraded second layer and replace it over healthier tissue.

But there are risks, including complete detachment of the retina, which occurs in about 25 percent of cases and can leave patients with poorer vision than when they started.

This is why companies like NeoStem are leading the way toward other treatments. In 2010, the company partnered with

187

Harvard's Schepens Eye Research Institute to test their very small embryonic-like (VSEL) cell technology for the treatment of macular degeneration. "Our research team is looking forward to leveraging our adult stem cell expertise to advance the understanding and development of very small embryonic-like stem cells for the treatment of age-related macular degeneration and glaucoma through our collaboration with the Schepens Institute," said Dr. Robin Smith, chairman and CEO of NeoStem, in a press release.

Another approach is that of Gabriel H. Travis, professor of ophthalmology and biological chemistry at the University of California, Los Angeles School of Medicine, who hopes to tap into the eye's existing stem cells. Unlike VSELs, these eye stem cells are difficult to harvest, and you get them in such sparse numbers that they require you to grow more in the lab (see chapter 14 about cancer treatments). But these existing eye stem cells are already "programmed" to do almost exactly what needs to be done, which is make retinal cells. Travis hopes to move the technology into clinical trial by 2014.

In 2010, Italian researchers chipped away at this cure by using stem cells to heal the eyes of people who had been blinded by chemical accidents. As always, this begins with a real story.

In 1994, twenty-four-year-old Damien Whitehall was riding a bus home from a night out in Newcastle, England. These late-night party buses have a reputation for being perhaps not the gentlest places, and on this night a fight broke out. Being an avid mountain biker and Jet Ski rider, Damien was strong and athletic. That night he stepped in to break up the fight, and one of the combatants took out a small bottle and sprayed him in the face with ammonia.

"As soon as the liquid hit me I was in agony. The pain was unbearable. I went to the hospital and was in there for two weeks.

When I was able to finally open my eye, I had lost just about all of my sight in it," Damien told the UK newspaper *Sun*. His cornea, the clear window at the front of the eye, was scarred and opaque.

The ammonia had killed the epithelium of Damien's cornea, the thin layer of cells that keeps the cornea clear. Remember how your eye is constantly renewing itself? Well, it's these limbal stem cells that do the renewing, spitting out a new outer layer of eye cells every day. Only in Damien's case, they couldn't. And so while macular degeneration is caused by the inability of a second layer of cells to perform their cleanup duties, Damien's chemical blindness was caused by the inability of his eye stem cells to maintain the essential layer that kept his cornea clear. Limbal stem cell deficiency leaves the eye cloudy and weeping, painfully sensitive to light, as if it were a raw wound that never heals.

Damien was in constant pain. Unable to drive, he lost his job. He also lost the ability to mountain bike and ride his Jet Ski. "I had years of treatment, but it was just trying different creams and ointments in a bid to stop the pain. None of them had any hope of restoring the sight," he told the *Sun*.

But there was an alternative. At a hospital near Whitehall in Newcastle, doctors sampled a tiny portion of the healthy limbal stem cells from Damien's left eye, from near where the colored part touches the white. They grew these stem cells in the lab and then layered them onto a tiny patch of amniotic sac material, donated after a baby's successful birth and which is commonly used for tissue engineering, because it nurtures growing tissue while remaining unlikely to be rejected by a patient's immune system. Surgeons then removed the dead tissue in Damien's right eye and stitched the new, stem-cell-rich tissue in its place.

"This has transformed my life," Damien told Mark Henderson, science editor of the *Times of London.* "My eye is almost as good as it was before the accident. I'm working, I can go Jet Skiing again, and I also ride horses. I have my life back thanks to the operation."

If this sounds like one of the many flukes you can find by surfing the Internet—one of the rare success stories in a sea of failures that go unreported—consider the fact that on July 8, 2010, the prestigious *New England Journal of Medicine* published Italian researchers' results of three- to ten-year follow-ups with 112 chemical or thermal burn patients who had undergone this surgery.

Of these 112 patients, the researchers wrote, "permanent restoration of a transparent, renewing corneal epithelium was attained in 76.6 percent of eyes." If the surgery failed, it did so right away, meaning that all 76.6 percent of the successful operations led to durable improvement. Of these 112 patients, three-quarters were cured. One patient who had been injured more than sixty years ago reported full recovery after the treatment.

The New York *Daily News* reported the reactions of stateside scientists who weren't involved with the study, including University of California ophthalmologist Ivan Schwab, who called the research "a roaring success," and Dr. Bruce Rosenthal, chief of low-vision programs at the vision-impairment nonprofit Lighthouse International, who said, "This is a major step in returning vision to someone who has lost it." Stem cells therefore give hope in curing burn blindness.

Similar corneal cloudiness affects about eight million people worldwide. While the current treatment relies on the existence of healthy limbal stem cells somewhere in an undamaged part of either eye, scientists hope to find deposits of similar enough stem cells elsewhere or learn to reprogram populations of skin stem cells into limbal stem cells, allowing patients with total blindness due to chemical or thermal cornea burns to undergo the procedure.

Sight isn't alone among the senses that might prove treatable with stem cells. Claude Monet went blind, but Beethoven went deaf. In 1824, after the premiere of his Ninth Symphony, friends had to turn Beethoven around to face the crowd so that he could notice their standing ovation. Hearing nothing, he wept.

Your inner ear works like wind blowing over a field of grain—tiny hairs ripple in the presence of vibrations, transmitting this information to nerve cells that connect to hearing centers in the brain. Historians debate the cause of Beethoven's deafness—was it lead poisoning, typhus, or maybe his habit of sticking his head in cold water to keep himself awake?—but the result was clear: by 1814 he was almost totally deaf. Whatever the cause, the tiny hairs in Beethoven's ears had been mown flat as surely as if a combine had harvested the crop. Because similar hearing loss can be caused by listening to music too loud, too long, many experts expect that as the iPod generation ages, the world may experience an epidemic of deafness like nothing it's seen before.

Luckily, almost exactly two hundred years after Beethoven went deaf, we're finally close to a cure. In April 2011, the journal *Stem Cells* reported the results of an Australian study that injected human olfactory stem cells into the inner ears of mice. As we've seen in other chapters, these olfactory stem cells are special—they're easy to harvest, and they're surprisingly multipotent, able to birth almost any tissue in the body, including heart cells, kidney cells, liver cells, muscle cells, and nerve cells.

But that's not what happened in the Australian study. Instead of becoming new hair cells in the organ of Corti in mice cochlea, these injected (human!) olfactory stem cells protected existing hair cells. If mice got stem cells in the very early stages of sensorineural hearing loss, they kept their hearing.

Researchers at Stanford took a step from protection toward a cure when they coaxed adult skin stem cells into making inner-ear hair cells in the lab. When they bent these hair cells with a thin spear of engineered glass, the cells shot electricity, just the way the natural cells do deep in the ear.

And so what we have is this: a proven stem cell cure for chemical- and burn-related blindness in one eye, a protection for the early stages of noise-related hearing loss pushing its way quickly into humans, and cures on the horizon for sensorineural hearing loss and dry macular degeneration.

Until the horizon comes into focus (pun intended), artist Virginia Doyle will have to continue doing what she can with what remains of her sight. She is legally blind, unable to drive, and without the ability to create art the way she has for forty years. But that doesn't mean she can't create art. As her disease has progressed, so has Virginia.

Before her condition, she was an Impressionist. In a 2008 exhibition in San Francisco's city hall, Virginia showed her new style. Her Abstract Expressionist painting *Family Stories II* is a tall, thin slice of color on canvas, with looping patterns of yellow, blue, green, and beige that run across the canvas like Arabic writing or graffiti. Virginia's new style is composed of patterns and images that are distinctly different from the way most people see the world—or, in Virginia's case, *don't* see the world.

When she was a sighted artist, "I was trying to be somebody else," she told the California Institute of Regenerative Medicine. Then when she lost her sight, "the real me came out, and I didn't care if I made mistakes." With the loss of her sight, Virginia's critical acclaim exploded.

Would you make the trade?

Chapter 17

HIV/AIDS

Sometimes serendipity is as powerful as science in curing disease. Such was the case when HIV-positive Timothy Ray Brown had a bone marrow transplant to cure leukemia. After doctors killed his cancerous blood system with chemotherapy and radiation and then replaced it with a bone marrow stem cell transplant from a matched adult donor, Timothy's leukemia went away...and so did his HIV. "I'm cured of HIV," he told CBS News in May 2011. "I had HIV, but I don't anymore." Living in Germany at the time of his treatment, Timothy was known as the "Berlin Patient" before going public—and his case is now one of the most famous in HIV/AIDS history.

The question is, what happened?

The human immunodeficiency virus—and, for that matter, any virus—is like a mosquito. It attaches to a cell and then inserts into the cell something a lot like a mosquito's proboscis. Only instead of extracting the cell's juice, a virus injects its own. The preferred prey of the HIV virus is the immune system's helper T cells, and when HIV catches one, it injects its own RNA into the T cell. The T cell weaves the HIV RNA into its own DNA, and from that point on, instead of going about its business of directing the immune system, the helper T cell has been "reprogrammed" to make copies of the HIV virus.

One thing that makes HIV so impossibly hard to cure is its ability to hide—to lie low inside the cells it's infected while the chemical warfare of treatment drugs rages on outside, only to go back into production once medication stops. HIV-positive patients on antiretroviral drugs can keep the disease at bay for years. But when these patients stop taking meds, the HIV RNA that's been spliced into helper T cells turns them back into little virus factories, spewing innumerable Xerox copies of HIV back into the body as if they were outlaws streaming from the cave where they've been hiding from the law.

And at that point the worst troubles start. The consequences can be dramatic. According to data published by the World Health Organization, "since the beginning of the epidemic, more than 60 million people have been infected with the HIV virus and nearly 30 million people have died of AIDS. In 2009, there were an estimated 33.3 million people living with HIV, 2.6 million new infections, and 1.8 million AIDS-related deaths. The WHO African Region is the most affected, where 1.8 million people acquired the virus in 2009. The estimated 1.3 million Africans who died of HIV-related illnesses in 2009 comprised 72 percent of the global total of 1.8 million deaths attributable to the epidemic."

There are many important links in the chain of the HIV life cycle, and researchers hope that by breaking one or more of these links, they'll be able to stop the progression of the disease. One promising link is the ability of HIV to get through the membrane of a helper T cell it's trying to infect. To do this, the HIV virus uses a protein called CCR5, which sits on the outside of helper T cells and functions like an open door. Everyone can make CCR5—the blueprints for this protein sit on chromosome number three—and though no one knows for sure, most scientists think it plays a minor role in the immune system's inflammatory response. In healthy humans, losing the protein isn't a big deal.

So as you can imagine, scientists have been working on drugs that nix this CCR5—without this protein, the HIV virus would be unable to invade helper T cells. But so far these "entry inhibitors" are proving pretty toxic, poisoning the liver as surely as they slam the door on HIV.

But there's another way to get rid of this protein CCR5, and that's to be born without the ability to make it. Some people have a little genetic mutation in chromosome number three. If both your mother and your father gave you chromosomes with this serendipitous defect, you won't be able to make CCR5. And this means you'll actually be immune to the HIV virus. About 20 percent of Caucasians get one faulty copy of the gene that makes CCR5, and about 1 percent gets two faulty copies and thus—as they would say on *Survivor*—the immunity idol.

The bone marrow donor who supplied the stem cells for Timothy Ray Brown's leukemia transplant was among this 1 percent holding the idol. The new stem cells that doctors infused into Timothy to cure his leukemia were genetically unable to make CCR5. And so when these stem cells churned out new helper T cells, HIV couldn't infect them.

On the CBS News video, forty-five-year-old Timothy is shown four years after his treatment, watering a large garden of potted plants outside his San Francisco home. He describes stopping his HIV antiretroviral medication the morning of his stem cell transplant . . . and not needing it since. CBS also interviewed Dr. Jay Levy, an AIDS researcher at the University of California, San Francisco who in 1983 codiscovered the AIDS virus. Instead of lucking into an HIV-immune donor, Levy imagines another way: "If you're able to take the white cells from someone and manipulate them so they're no longer infectable by HIV and those white cells become the whole immune system of that individual, you've got essentially what we call a functional cure."

Timothy Ray Brown was the first person cured of HIV in world history.

There are a couple of things standing in the way of bone marrow stem cell transplants becoming the widely used treatment for HIV. The first is the extreme risk of bone marrow transplant in general. Without transplant, leukemia patients would be expected to die within the year, and so in the case of leukemia, drastic times call for the drastic measure of a bone marrow transplant. But in HIV, antiretroviral medications and other drugs can extend a patient's years of quality life past the point that the risks of a bone marrow transplant would be a viable trade.

The second difficulty in bone marrow transplants as a cure for HIV is the difficulty of finding a bone marrow donor who is both a genetic match and among the 1 percent who are immune to HIV. It's hard enough to find a matched donor, let alone the *fifty* matched donors that make one donor's immunity to HIV more than 50 percent likely.

To solve this second problem, the company Sangamo BioSciences showed that it takes a thief to catch a thief. Do you remember how HIV works by inserting its own code into the DNA of helper T cells? Well, Sangamo engineered a way to get to these cells first, snipping their DNA in a way that disabled their ability to make the protein CCR5 that HIV needs to get inside. Again, taking away this protein is like slamming the door in HIV's face. The technique works by using something called a zinc-finger nuclease, which can be designed to recognize any sequence of DNA. When a zinc-finger nuclease recognizes the right pattern, it uses its "fingers" to pull it out of the genetic code—in other words, it's a way to snip a specific gene.

Working with HIV patients whose immune systems remained low despite treatment with the standard antiretroviral cocktails, Sangamo harvested patients' helper T cells, used a zinc-finger nuclease to snip the gene that makes CCR5 (the door), and then injected these modified cells back into patients. On September 18, 2011, the company presented the results of its clinical trial of their gene-therapy door-locking strategy at the fifty-first annual Interscience Conference on Antimicrobial Agents and Chemotherapy in Chicago. As reported in *Discover* magazine and many other news outlets, in most of the fifteen patients treated, these engineered cells didn't survive once they were injected (scientists don't know why). But in two patients, HIV levels dropped tenfold, and in one patient, HIV dropped to undetectable levels.

This is gene therapy, and it's very, very special.

Still, it's even more fascinating when combined with stem cell technologies, and this is exactly what researchers at the California Institute for Regenerative Medicine are doing. Introducing genetic resistance to a regular helper T cell makes that cell immune to HIV. But eventually, no matter how many HIV-immune helper T cells you inject into a patient, they die out, and HIV is presented with a new crop of naïve targets. But if you introduce this genetic resistance into the bone marrow stem cells themselves, then every helper T cell these stem cells birth will inherit this resistance. Instead of using zinc-finger nucleases to genetically modify helper T cells, researchers at CIRM are doing the same thing to the blood stem cells that parent them.

It goes even a step further.

Imagine that in your bone marrow are stem cells that have

been engineered to be HIV resistant along with your original stem cells that remain susceptible. Eventually HIV kills these susceptible stem cells, leaving *only the resistant cells*. So, ironically and fittingly, HIV contributes to its own demise. In a blood system in which even a few of the bone marrow stem cells are resistant, over time the virus kills all of its nonresistant prey, leaving itself with no susceptible cells to convert into HIV factories, and so the virus eventually dies off.

A press release from CIRM calls this "cellular jujitsu," turning the killing power of HIV against itself. The press release says, "Whereas other genetic engineering approaches must alter great numbers of cells to create lasting change, and must keep those new cells running for a lifetime, the jujitsu nature of the zinc-finger approach means the zinc fingers must operate only briefly, mutating only a small percentage of all the stem cells." After that, it's survival of the fittest, and unfortunately for HIV, the fittest stem cells are the ones it can't infect.

Dr. John Zaia, who pioneered this approach as the Aaron D. and Edith Miller Endowed Chair in Gene Therapy at City of Hope Hospital, expects to move the zinc-finger nuclease approach of snipping the CCR5 gene from HIV patients' stem cells into clinical trials soon.

If you understood that thick sentence, you're doing well. And we assure you it's worth it to keep reading. The following is a less pacifistic approach to stem cell treatment of HIV—instead of using gene therapy to make cells resistant to HIV, researchers at UCLA hope to use similar therapy to engineer cells that kill the virus itself.

"There are two types of T-cells—CD4 [helper] and CD8 [killer] cells," says Jerome Zack, PhD, professor of microbiology, in an interview with the California Institute for Regenerative Medicine. "CD4 cells are the ones that get infected; CD8 cells are the ones that kill infected cells and stop virus replication. What we're doing is engineering the stem cell to become a CD8 killer cell that could actually kill HIV-infected T-cells."

In fact, a few of an HIV patient's killer T cells already have the ability to recognize and destroy cells infected by the HIV virus. Like developing resistance to any virus, these killer T cells program themselves by manufacturing a protein that they stick on their outer cell wall, like a pirate flag that describes the kind of gold-laden ship they're looking to plunder. Only, unfortunately, there aren't enough of these HIV-specific pirates in the body to win the war against the massive armada that is HIV.

So Zack and his team decided it would be a good idea to make more.

He harvested these killer Ts that could target HIV, grew the "receptor" that allows killer Ts to recognize the virus, and then used some nifty genetic engineering to insert the blueprints for this receptor into blood stem cells.

When they inserted these engineered stem cells into mice, the stem cells churned out killer T cells—in this case killer Ts complete with the pirate-flag protein they needed to target cells infected with the HIV virus. These cells were armed to search and destroy, and what they specifically wanted to destroy was HIV.

"What we're really doing is engineering the immune system using genetic engineering to respond to a foreign particle of choice, in this case, the AIDS virus," Zack says. "Basically, we've shown that you can engineer the immune system in humans to fight whatever infection you'd like, so we're now also moving forward towards using this technique to fight cancer or other viral infections."

Take a second, because that's astounding: this promising stem cell cure for HIV/AIDS may, in fact, point the way toward the cure of viral infections *in general*.

Zack says, "Clearly, for regenerative medicine, for fighting many diseases, including infectious diseases like we're proposing, stem cells really are, in my opinion, the way of the future."

Chapter 18

How to Find Safe Stem Cell Therapies

When Bernie van Zyl was diagnosed with a then-untreatable form of degenerative heart disease, he went on the offensive, tracking down an early clinical trial for a stem cell therapy that saved his life. He wrote, "My experience illustrates that seriously ill and dying patients can take charge of their own cases and be certain they are receiving the best possible treatment."

Volunteer firefighter Zack Michaels raised funds for treatment in Tijuana with stem cell injections that he credits with his partial recovery from traumatic brain injury.

How can you, like Bernie, enroll in a hopeful clinical trial that jumps past what's even considered cutting edge? Is medical tourism like Zack's ever the answer? It raises more concerns than each of us singularly can imagine. We want you to be aware of risks related to those treatments that claim miraculous results without strong scientific evidence.

Keep reading.

In fact, there are only two distinct ways to find valuable stem cell treatments. The gold standard of proven effectiveness and safety are treatments based on well-performed and documented research that consequently leads the United States Food and

Drug Administration (or similar governmental agencies in other countries) to approve them for medical treatment. The next best option is treatments that are in the FDA approval process, meaning stem cell therapies that are currently in clinical trials.

Of course, some would say that outside these trials, you may still be able to pay out of pocket for some types of stem cell treatments offered at clinics in the United States, or even to explore medical tourism at research universities around the world. For many reasons, these solutions represent significant risk that we also want to bring to your attention.

FDA-Approved Treatments

Some stem cell treatments are FDA-approved and widely available at hospitals throughout the United States. Of the many advantages of FDA-approved treatments, a big one is cost—if an FDA-approved treatment matches your condition, your medical insurance should pay for it. While health insurances may differ, the standard workflow for getting any specialized treatment starts with your general practitioner, who can refer you to a specialist, who may refer you to another specialist or may troubleshoot your treatment him- or herself. Specialists should work with you to choose FDA-approved stem cell treatments and should work with your insurance company to ensure they're covered.

That said, after reading this book or researching a condition online, you may learn of FDA-approved stem cell treatments that your general practitioner hasn't mentioned or maybe hasn't even heard of. In that case, if you've discovered the name of a promising drug, for example, a good first step is a visit to the FDA database of approved drugs, which you can find with a quick Internet search for *Drugs@FDA*. Type in the name of the drug you're interested in to discover whether it is, in fact, approved. Then, don't be afraid to bring up specific treatments with your doctors.

Common conditions treated by FDA-approved stem cell treatments include leukemia and sickle cell anemia. It's very likely that a host of other diseases of the blood and immune system will soon join this list, and it's also very likely that stem cell treatments for burns, tendon injuries, and heart diseases will join the list by the end of 2014.

Stem Cell Treatments in FDA-Approved Clinical Trials

This category includes the bulk of the treatments mentioned in this book. Start by talking to a specialist, who should be up-to-date on clinical trials that match your condition or at least on the condition-specific resources that you can use to quickly and easily find relevant clinical trials.

That said—unfortunately!—for this and the following three flavors of stem cell treatments, you may have to be your own expert and advocate. Clinical trials are at the cutting edge, and even the best-trained doctor may not be able to stay on top of each and every stem cell treatment in the trials pipeline. The simple truth is that you are almost certainly more motivated to find a trial than your specialist. And this motivation can lead to finding the overlooked stem cell diamond in the rough that has an outside chance of helping or healing your condition.

Start by learning as much as you can about your condition. Write down what you know and then visit ClinicalTrials.gov. This website is a one-stop database for absolutely every clinical trial approved by the FDA. But because ClinicalTrials.gov collects everything, the information you find there can be overwhelming. For example, in the fall of 2011, typing *leukemia* into the search box returned 3,767 results. But adding *stem cells* to the list cuts it down to 1,379, and adding *acute myeloid* to *leukemia* cuts it down to 583. Further refining this search by clicking the box for only open studies cuts the list down to 232. This is a manageable number. And if you like, you can display these clinical trials on a map, discovering which trials are nearby.

That said, one nice thing about clinical trials is that it may not matter where the trial is located. Many trials reimburse for travel expenses, and the $1,000 that might be dear to you is a drop in the bucket of the $100 million or so a drug company may pay to take a drug from research to approval.

Another powerful feature of ClinicalTrials.gov is the ability to browse by disease type. This is especially helpful in finding stem cell trials, because many stem cell studies don't have "stem cell" in the title. The website ClinicalConnection.com is a nongovernmental option for running similar searches and offers the ability to set up alerts that will notify you when new trials matching your criteria become available.

Still, searching these databases can be overwhelming. According to the Center for Information and Study of Clinical Research Participation, in 2007 more than 26,000 researchers were involved in running clinical trials. That's a lot of trials, and sifting through ClinicalTrials.gov or ClinicalConnection.com for a stem cell trial that matches your condition can be daunting, to say the least.

Instead, you might try starting with the websites of organizations that have already done this sifting for you. Research associations are a good place to go. For example, the American Association for Cancer Research (http://aacr.org) includes a section titled "Survivors and Advocates," where you'll find information on support groups, financial aid, and clinical trials. Included on the AACR "How to Find a Clinical Trial" page are various phone numbers and links to websites that will accept your medical information and match you with relevant trials. For example, the AACR points to the website http://breastcancertrials.org, which walks breast cancer patients through a step-by-step process of finding matching clinical trials.

The American Diabetes Association (http://www.diabetes.org) has a similar clinical trials matching page under its "News and Research" tab. Similarly, the Juvenile Diabetes Research Foundation (http://jdrf.org), a big advocate for stem cell research, has a clinical trials page under their "Research" tab. The same is true of the National Stroke Association (http://www.stroke.org), the American Heart Association (http://www.heart.org), the American Autoimmune Related Diseases Association (http://www.aarda.org), and many, many others.

If you get frustrated, consider contacting these associations directly. Many will be able to direct you over the phone to promising clinical trials.

Only as a last resort and if you have ample time should you look for clinical trial information in message boards for patients with your disease. Though usually posted with the best of intentions, the reality is that much of the information submitted by other patients is outdated or mistaken. Worse yet, some of these "patients" contributing their stories are in fact hucksters posing as patients to promote their products. On the Internet, you just don't know who's on the other end of a post. These message boards and patient forums may be a good source of support and inspiration, but for information on clinical trials, it's usually more useful (and safer) to stick to government and reputable association sources.

Once you find a clinical trial that looks like a match for your condition, get in touch with the study coordinator. Near the bottom of every ClinicalTrials.gov listing is a section titled "Contact and Locations," which should include phone numbers and e-mail addresses for clinical trial administrators. Don't be afraid—get in touch. These administrators need you, the patient, and so should be willing to walk you through any and all of the next steps. And if it turns out you're not a match after all, as happens in many cases, ask for related trials that may be more appropriate for you; they often know of related trials for which you may qualify.

It's a call that could save your life.

FDA-Approved Clinical Trials Outside the United States

The United States is certainly not the only country in the world doing good science. And, perhaps surprisingly, the FDA doesn't only oversee clinical trials in the United States.

Instead, a January 2011 article in *Vanity Fair* points out that in 1998, 271 FDA clinical trials were registered outside the United States, and in 2008 that number had risen to 6,485, with similar exponential growth expected to continue. In the fall of 2011, a quick search on ClinicalTrials.gov showed 1,190 clinical trials in China alone that were actively recruiting participants. Narrowing this to stem cell trials returned active studies for cirrhosis, diabetic foot, spinal cord injury, stroke, diabetes, Parkinson's, burns, anemia, ataxia, neuromyelitis optica, lupus, and a variety of musculoskeletal conditions—sixty-three active stem cell studies in all. Brazil had seventeen open, FDA-approved stem cell clinical trials, India had eight, and Russia had ten. Again, these numbers are only likely to rise.

Perhaps cynically, the *Vanity Fair* article describes the appeal to big drug companies of these overseas trials:

It's cheaper to run trials in places where the local population survives on only a few dollars a day. It's also easier to recruit patients, who often believe they are being treated for a disease rather than, as may be the case, just getting a placebo as part of an experiment. And it's easier to find what the industry calls "drug-naïve" patients: people who are not being treated for any disease and are not currently taking any drugs and indeed may never have taken any—the sort of people who will almost certainly yield better test results. Regulations in many foreign countries are also less stringent, if there are any regulations at all. The risk of litigation is negligible, in some places nonexistent. Finally—a significant plus for the drug companies—the FDA does so little monitoring that the companies can pretty much do and say what they want.

The rest of the article, which you can find with a quick Internet search for the name of the magazine and the title of the article, "Deadly Medicine," is certainly worth reading. Many other sources come to similar conclusions: the world of non-US clinical trials would benefit from tighter controls. And it doesn't take long to turn up a plethora of horror stories of patients who have been harmed by experimental medicines.

But what if the flip side is also true? Might these trials also be distancing patients in the United States from the newest, brightest stem cell treatments?

While it's not unheard of for an American to take part in a foreign clinical trial, many hurdles stand in the way. First, clinical trials don't accept just anybody—there are many criteria that trial patients must meet. If an American does not meet the criteria for a Russian clinical trial, the logistics are daunting, to say the least. Most trials require prescreening, testing, and multiple follow-up visits, which mean repeated trips to the research site. Many clinical trials do help cover patients' travel costs within reason—but unfortunately, international travel is unlikely to be within reason.

Non-FDA-Approved Treatments Offered in United States Clinics

In this book, you learned about Texas governor Rick Perry's stem cell treatment as part of spinal fusion surgery. You heard about pitcher Bartolo Colón, who had stem cells injected into his torn rotator cuff. And you heard about the Centeno-Schultz clinic in Broomfield, Colorado, that now offers same-day therapies in the United States and mesenchymal stem cell injections in the Cayman Islands to combat a range of sports injuries and conditions like arthritis.

The stem cells used in these therapies were once believed by the practitioners to fall into the category of "minimally manipulated" cell products and thus were permissible under FDA guidelines as tissues (HCT/P, 21 CFR 1271). Regulators disagreed with this categorization and, in addition, have indicated that the cell products are not considered tissues according to the "homologous use" exemption, meaning that the agency considers the manipulated cells as not being used for the same purpose as the particular stem cells from which they were originally derived. For both of these reasons, they are regulated differently than tissues and therefore require clinical trials and FDA approval of a biologic license application (BLA) before being commercially sold and allowed to become standard of care in the United States.

Still, a June 2011 *USA Today* article titled "Unapproved Stem Cell Treatments Causing Concern" quotes George Daley, director of stem cell transplantation research at Children's Hospital Boston, as saying, "Lots of patients have been harmed by otherwise well-intentioned but misinformed practitioners."

When you step off the path of FDA-approved treatments, you officially enter the Wild West of medical care. Some of these treatments very likely work. Some of them almost certainly don't. For example, the more than two hundred patients treated for musculoskeletal problems at the Centeno-Schultz Clinic coupled with the proven success of nearly identical treatments in racehorses provides extremely compelling evidence for the effectiveness of these treatments (whose results are likely to be published in the near future). But elsewhere, for every Bartolo Colón whose miracle comeback may have been fueled by stem cell injections, there is a Peyton Manning, the former Indianapolis Colts star quarterback who flew to Europe for stem cell injections into his ailing neck before the 2011–2012 football season and who nevertheless had to follow this failed procedure with a season-ending neck surgery.

The International Cellular Medicine Society (http://cellmedicinesociety.org) offers information that sits on either side of this fence. The organization writes that it "represents over 1,000 physicians, researchers and patients from over 35 countries on 6 continents." And the website of the ICMS is one-stop shopping for stem cell treatments from both the doctor and patient perspectives, offering links to the latest research, clinical guidelines for the harvesting and use of stem cells, patient forums attesting to the power of stem cells, an annual conference, and even certification for clinics that offer stem cell therapies.

Many of the ICMS activities seem to be very honest attempts to ensure quality care and provide both doctors and patients with needed information and resources, including published standards for the use of patient claims that state, "Clinics that seek to position cell based medical treatments as a 'miracle product' and/or claim to cure serious conditions are not credible, pose a significant risk to public health and safety and are not acceptable practices." The research section of the ICMS website points to the latest PubMed articles for many of the conditions described in this book.

Bravo.

But despite the regulation of clinical best practices and the attempt to reign in rampant, unfounded claims of miracle cures, it's also a bit unclear where the ICMS draws the line between (nearly proven) effective treatments in places like the Centeno-Schultz Clinic and clinics offering (extremely unproven) stem cell treatments for conditions like cerebral palsy, epilepsy, autism, spinal cord injury, and Lou Gehrig's disease.

Notice this fine line: it's very likely that the invasive and dangerous therapy of immune system suppression followed by bone marrow transplant will make its way from FDA-approved clinical trials into clinics for the treatment of Lou Gehrig's disease. But it's unlikely that the clinics currently offering infusions of an ALS patient's stem cells are doing much good. Though both are tagged with "stem cell treatment for ALS," these are very different procedures with very different likely results—and it shows the difference between a research hospital and a private clinic.

Yes, the certification of stem cell clinics can help ensure conformity to safety standards. No, conforming to these safety standards doesn't imply that the treatments of every certified clinic are effective. Again, it's an industry in which it's almost impossible to pin down what works and what doesn't yet work—and there's an ever-moving fence that divides real treatments from shams.

And so many hard-and-fast rules aren't hard and fast. That said, here is this book's best attempt at a hard-and-fast rule (irony intended): improvement in musculoskeletal injuries and other conditions can come from clinics, but "miracle" cures almost exclusively come from the US FDA-approved treatments and clinical trials described previously.

You may find exceptions to this rule. But your best chances for success lie along the same paths as the people in this book who pursued FDA-approved trials and treatments—journeys of hope, of progress, and of cures.

Remember, legitimate scientific research is not the purview of private opinion or personal viewpoint. It is a matter of accepted practices and well-documented results, openly available to the international scientific community for evaluation, replication, and improvement. When scientific inquiry is combined with high ethical values, it serves society best of all. This applies especially to adult stem cell research, which holds such tremendous promise to treat illness and alleviate suffering around the world.

For reliable information on current developments in adult stem cell research, as well as information on our unique partnership with the Vatican to explore the cultural, ethical, and human implications of adult stem cell use, please visit our website at the Stem for Life Foundation.

Acknowledgments

The authors would like to make a special acknowledgment to Dr. W. E. Bosarge and his Bosarge Family Foundation for their unwavering support of adult stem cell research. His dedication to medicine worldwide is greatly valued and respected, and we all applaud his generosity and commitment to further science and innovation. A special thank-you to Garth Sundem, Jon Ford, Jan Miller, Matthew Henninger, Eric Powers, and Martin Schmieg for their assistance in creating this guide to educate people around the world regarding the potential for stem cells to save lives and decrease human suffering.

Advil® is a registered trademark of Wyeth LLC.

Avastin® is a registered trademark of Genentech Inc.

Avonex® is a registered trademark of Biogen Idec MA Inc.

Band-Aid® is a registered trademark of Johnson & Johnson Corp.

Baskin-Robbins® is a registered trademark of BR IP Holder LLC.

Botox® is a registered trademark of Allergan Inc.

ELA® cells is a registered trademark of Parcell Laboratories LLC.

Erbitux® is a registered trademark of ImClone LLC.

Google™ is a registered trademark of Google Technology Inc.

hLEC™ is a trademark of StemCells Inc.

iPod® is a registered trademark of Apple Inc.

J.Crew® is a registered trademark of J. Crew International Inc.

Jet Ski® is a registered trademark of Kawasaki Heavy Industries Ltd.

M&M's® is a registered trademark of Mars Inc.

Mitsubishi® is a registered trademark of Mitsubishi Motors Corp.

Nautilus® is a registered tradement of Nautilus Inc.

Neupogen® is a registered trademark of Amgen Inc.

ReCell® is a registered trademark of C3 Operations Pty Ltd.

Regenexx® is a registered trademark of Regenerative Sciences LLC.

Sinemet® is a registered trademark of Merck Sharp & Dohme Corp.

Solu-Medrol® is a registered trademark of Pharmacia & Upjohn Company LLC.

TiLite® is a registered trademark of TiSport LLC.

Tupperware® is a registered trademark of Dart Industries Inc.

Twinkies® is a registered trademark of Hostess Brands Inc.

Xerox® is a registered trademark of Xerox Corp.